BOOKS, MANUSCRIPTS, and THE HISTORY OF MEDICINE

BOOKS, MANUSCRIPTS, and THE HISTORY OF MEDICINE

Essays on the Fiftieth Anniversary of the Osler Library

edited by PHILIP M. TEIGEN

Science History Publications

New York — 1982

Published by Science History Publications/USA
a division of
Neale Watson Academic Publications, Inc.
156 Fifth Avenue, New York, NY 10010

Library of Congress Cataloging in Publication Data
Main entry under title:

Books, manuscripts, and the history of medicine.

Includes bibliographical references and index.
Contents: Introduction / Lloyd G. Stevenson — "Dry,
dusty, tedious, accursed, hateful bibliography" :
Osler and British bibliography / Charles G. Roland —
Medical-historical research in mediaeval and Renaissance
manuscripts / Richard J. Durling — [etc.]
1. Medicine—Bibliography—History—Addresses, essays,
lectures.   2. Medicine—Bibliography—Theory, methods,
etc.—Addresses, essays, lectures.   3. Medical literature
—History—Addresses, essays, lectures.   4. Medicine—
Historiography—Addresses, essays, lectures.
5. Osler Library—Addresses, essays, lectures.
I. Teigen, Philip M.   II. Osler Library.
Z6659.5.B66   [R118.6]   010   82-5739
ISBN 0-88202-199-0   AACR2

Publication of this book has been made possible by a grant from the Associated Medical
Services, Inc. and the Hannah Institute for the History of Medicine.

Designed and manufactured in the U.S.A.

Acknowledgments

The essays in this book were prepared for a symposium commemorating the fiftieth anniversary of the Osler Library. Since Sir William Osler successfully united—as few others have done—interests in libraries, bibliography, and the history of medicine, the fiftieth anniversary of the reception of his library at McGill University seemed an appropriate occasion on which to examine the ways the history of medicine, librarianship, and bibliography still occupy common ground. Towards this end, in preparing their papers, the five contributors reviewed, among other things, the past fifty to seventy-five years of research in their respective fields of scholarship. This seemed a useful way of introducing the audience to unfamiliar subject areas and of providing an opportunity for scholars to examine historically their own disciplines. This latter approach is, I believe, an essential heuristic procedure for practising historians and bibliographers, as well as for librarians, the discipline of the last group being one that is based on both managerial and technological understanding.

Thanks go first to the five essayists who communicated their special knowledge to an audience not as familiar with it and to the moderator who contributed an introduction to this collection. Second, I thank the several agencies that supported the symposium financially: the Hannah Institute for the History of Medicine, Toronto; the Social Science and Humanities Research Council of Canada; the University Library System, McGill University; the Faculty of Graduate Studies and Research, McGill University; and the Friends of the Osler Library.

In helping to prepare these essays for publication, David A.E. Shephard contributed invaluable assistance as reader, collaborator, and editorial advisor; Carolyn Kato provided the necessary typing; and Mrs. Karin-Maria Waterhouse looked after a host of details throughout the symposium itself as well as during its planning.

Philip M. Teigen
Osler Librarian

Contents

Introduction

Lloyd G. Stevenson

Lloyd G. Stevenson

The fiftieth birthday of the Osler Library of McGill University (29 May 1979) comes when bibliography, as a means of access to the ever burgeoning medical literature, has passed far beyond the century-old *Index Medicus* (discontinued a generation ago) and has entered fully into the electronic age. Medical bibliography in fact has led the way, its terminals flashing with the lights of a new era. This is enumerative bibliography, classified and arranged, and poised to give answers to today's pressing questions; but it is capable of serving many needs in many ways. Among *The Great Medical Bibliographers* considered by Fulton in his book of that name are a majority of bibliographers—Gesner, Haller, Ploucquet, Billings are examples—whose aims were practical and who had something in common not only with Osler, Cushing and Fulton but also with Frank B. Rogers, he of MEDLARS, and with the electronic revolution of the late twentieth century.

In bibliography of other kinds—the evaluative, historical kinds, of which some were those well known to William Osler and to William Willoughby Francis—literature has long taken the lead and the pace has been more decorous. The advance has been steady nevertheless; it began early and it continues through delectable valleys and sunny uplands. To give some account of its progress (in the context but generally not with the aid, of computerized bibliography) was the purpose of the five bibliographers, librarians and historians who on a momentous day spoke about *Books, Manuscripts, and the History of Medicine.* They were looking, as historians, to the past, but we learn from them how they are bringing novel techniques to the aid of critical bibliography and how they are looking, with curbed but unshaken confidence, to the future.

One speaker from Canada, two from the United States, one from Germany and one from England, were gently mustered by the chairman, a Canadian long resident in the U.S.A. and to be filed, so to speak, on a green card. The international character of the panel was fitting to the occasion and to the memory of William Osler, who may perhaps be said to have spent the second half of his life, the last thirty-five years, in travelling abroad. His books, of course, returned to Montreal, and here, ten years after his death, having been equipped meanwhile with a magnificent catalogue, the *Bibliotheca Osleriana*, they were installed.

Throughout a rewarding day the new electronic bibliography was quite properly a minor theme. The day began with Charles Roland's appropriate review of the bibliographical interests of Sir William Osler and his relations with the British bibliography of his time. From a learned survey by Richard Durling of medical-historical research in mediaeval and renaissance manuscripts to an interesting and very knowledgeable account by Thomas Tanselle of physical bibliography in the twentieth century, the emphasis lay on the extension of aims and techniques that would both have been seen as altogether conversable by the men from whom Osler, during the last chapter of his life, learned the pleasures of expert bibliography. Estelle Brodman lamented the present lack of evaluative bibliographers in the Osler-Cushing-Fulton-Keynes tradition and looked "forward into historical medical bibliography" with the possibility of computer help. Eric Freeman adumbrated "a social history of the medical book," feeling that neither this nor social medical history more generally need be incompatible with analytical bibliography and textual studies: it might be accomplished, he concluded sadly, "if only the historians would re-order some of their priorities." The medical book as a physical object and as a social phenomenon seemed to almost all the participants, however, to have had too little notice; presumably attention has been focussed too exclusively, in their view, on the text. On the other hand, they deplored any departure from evaluative work and in fact demonstrated how their methods may, and do, contribute to textual studies. The spokesman for physical bibliography in the twentieth century—Tanselle—had, as a matter of fact, some of the best things to say about the interpretation of text.

A bibliographer who is concerned above all with descriptive or physical bibliography and who is ready to push his art and science beyond the merely esthetic, the caressing description of beautiful books, has much in common with the archeologist, with the numismatist and more directly, of course, with the paleographer. He can induce the matter under his hands to reveal secrets, the substantial to substantiate or disprove. He combines the functions of detective and barrister. Not only can Elizabethan spelling be a literary and bibliographic clue but headlines can be bibliographic evidence; half-sheet imposition can tell the whole story, plate damage make a case. Tanselle assures us that "the bibliographical and editorial scholarship directed toward belletristic texts will eventually be applied to all kinds of texts, and the sooner this expansion takes place the better for everyone concerned." Nor need we question this further dictum: "Although Sir William Osler would probably not be drawn to some of the tasks now incumbent on

4

bibliographers, he would unquestionably be in sympathy with the larger ends to be achieved by bibliographical cooperation among those working in different fields." Especially is this so because, as demonstrated in Tanselle's essay, the methods of descriptive bibliography, already helpful in settling certain questions of priority, also promise to be of importance to the very meaning of scientific texts. These and other services already familiar are to be added to those long expected and required by the collector.

(The continuing extension to science and medicine of what were in origin belletristic methods in bibliography will repay in some measure the gift of the electronic procedures first developed, to the point of being brought into service, in the medical sphere—computerized information retrieval begins with MEDLARS—and now being extended more and more into other areas, even so far as the belletristic.)

What does bibliography actually do, pragmatic scholars may ask, for history or for literature? To this guileless question the dedicated bibliographers of sixteenth- and seventeenth-century drama perhaps supply the most nearly probative answer, but it is one that is now almost matched in a great many other, including twentieth-century, domains. From participants in the Osler symposium we have heard as much about literature as about medicine and science. It is in the fields of literature that bibliography has grown and matured. But it is obvious that in no field, not even in Shakespearean bibliography serving drama, can it rival the function of physiology in relation to medicine; and yet modern analytical bibliography is unquestionably a "literary science" serving literature and an "historical science" serving history much as physiology is a medical science. The degree of history's dependence on bibliography we need not specify; it varies enormously with the kind and the period of history.

In what sense, then, is bibliography a discrete science, something sufficient unto itself? In one sense certainly; in other senses possibly. When they write or speak of historical bibliography, the experts do not mean, as above, a science in the service of history but a science making use of a special kind of history—the study, usually highly technical, of the development of book production and publication. Textual bibliography, or the detailed study of the material form with the object of discovering the authentic text and its history through examination of the circumstances of publication, is not the same thing: it is obviously dependent on historical bibliography, as just defined, and may be seen as an extension of it, but it obviously requires additional resources. Pollard was a superb analytical textual bibliographer because he had two strings to his bow: he was very learned in the history of book production and publication and at the same time he was a fine literary scholar, profoundly learned in the dramatic literature of his period. If the second kind of expertise, the analytical textual, is the more impressive of the two it is only to the degree in which two high skills or proficiencies are combined to cardinal effect. Had Pollard attempted, as he certainly would not have done, to use his wonderful historical knowledge of book production and publication to study the developing literature of early chemistry, he would have lost his extraordinary dual advantage; he would have fallen a little bit short of the highest standard of autonomous professional bibliography. "Again and again," declares Cowley, "the most expert bibliographical workers have insisted that subject knowledge must precede bibliography"—a point he illustrates with quotations from Greg, Esdaile and Pollard. Said Pollard: "The chemist must make his own bibliography of chemistry, for he, and he only, possesses the knowledge of the subject which can make such a bibliography intelligent."

This brings us to what is the most widely practiced kind of bibliography and the kind least likely to be considered in the light of an art or a science—subject bibliography or the cataloguing and description of material as a preliminary to the study of the subject. This is probably the bibliographic art most directly useful to medicine and it is now an art of venerable age. Gesner, at the time of his death (1565), had not completed the subject classification for medicine and surgery which he had projected but others began within a generation to make attempts. Of these the earliest was the work of Israel Spach, whose *Nomenclator Scriptorum Medicorum* was published at Frankfort in 1591, enumerating 1,436 medical writers classified under some thirty subject groupings. Ploucquet, Forbes, Callisen and Billings bring the story forward to the foundation of the *Index-Catalogue* a little more than a century ago. A great chapter then begins which did not end until 1950 when, in the middle of the letter M of the fourth series, "the greatest bibliographical tool that has ever been created for the medical profession of the world" was discontinued, "smothered by its own weight." The age of MEDLARS was not far off, HISTLINE only a little farther. The latter is potentially of great use to medical historians in its singular way but it is a doorway to the past that will not be wide open until well into the future. Meantime, to some degree like the comparable but much larger and more urgent services which encompass the seething present, it is open and doing business.

It is a major theme of Eric Freeman in his stimulating contribution to this fiftieth-anniversary symposium that medical historians, libraries and bibliographers might much better profit from each other's skills and insights. This symposium is in itself a subscription to that cause and ought, indeed, to move it forward. A splendid example, from Montreal, of the joyous cooperative effort in scholarship in which such skills and insights can be harnessed is the Tercentenary Edition (1664-1964) of *The Anatomy of the Brain and Nerves* by Thomas Willis which William Feindel edited in 1965 and which includes, along with his own fine essay on the origin and significance of the book, "A Bibliographic Survey of *Cerebri Anatome*" by H.R. Denham, a comprehensive and meticulous work which will stand as a beacon in Willis studies. How it would have delighted Osler we need little imagination to guess.

Only in the first year of the First World War did Geoffrey Keynes issue the first of the many examples of the personal bibliography with which his name will always be linked, for he is credited with having pioneered the form; and Osler had been gone for five years when Keynes produced *A Bibliography of Sir Thomas Browne*, one that Osler would have valued far above all others.

It was the belief of Professor Fulton that "the bibliographies of most enduring value are those prepared by men who have approached their task with the utilitarian and the humanistic viewpoints in equitable balance." That neither the utmost refinements of technology in the sphere of physical bibliography nor the enormous, the magical comprehension and discrimination of the electronic enumerators will shoulder aside personal bibliography (Janet Doe's *Paré*, William Lefanu's *Jenner*, Keynes' *Browne*, *Hook* and *Harvey* and Fulton's splendid *Boyle*) with other examples of critical, evaluative bibliography is devoutly to be wished. The fiftieth anniversary of the opening of the Osler Library has witnessed heartening examples of that equipoise between the utilitarian and the cultural which will maintain the warm familiar spirit of medical bibliography, however much the new potentialities change and expand it and extend its uses. Osler would have recognized as friends and colleagues the five who spoke on the great day.

7

"Dry, Dusty, Tedious, Accursed, Hateful, Bibliography": Osler and British Bibliography

Charles G. Roland

The bibliographic activities of Osler, although not virgin territory, have been less ploughed than many other Oslerian fields. My paper concerns these activities, particularly during the last 14 years of his life—the Oxford years, 1905 to 1919.

Bibliography Defined and Osler's Approach to Bibliography

No definition of the word *bibliography* is both comprehensive and succinct. The question of a definition has long been debated, many of the prominent of those who contributed to the debate being bibliographers who were friends or acquaintances of William Osler. The problem in arriving at a satisfactory definition was characterized by Fredson Bowers, who wrote that the word *bibliography* has had many meanings subsuming "too many activities to be very exact in definition."[1] Walter W. Greg defined the word to mean "the study of books as material objects,"[2] and stated that "bibliography has nothing to do with the subject or literary content of the book."[3]

And there is the rock upon which most definitions founder. Those who speak for the profession of bibliography have attempted to exorcise content, and, though many bibliographies continue to have much to do with content, current definitions do exclude it. Bowers divided bibliography into enumerative and analytical types, and further divided analytical into descriptive and textual.[4] On the use of formalized analytical bibliography he wrote as follows:

> Physical evidence gained from identifying hundreds of pieces of slightly bent or broken type, and from following them in and out of the printers' cases as they were typeset, distributed, and typeset again in different family groups on various pages, enabled C.J.K. Hinman to establish the fact that the Shakespeare First Folio was not composed and printed in normal order but instead in a leapfrog manner. [Ultimately] . . . not only the workman who set the type but the order of composition of each page and the order in which it went through the press can now be determined for English literature's most important single book.[5]

This is bibliography at a highly rarified level; it may give some impression of the power and the intellectual utility of the science of bibliography. But it is not Osler's type of bibliography: Osler could not separate the study of the physical book from the study of its content, and he was far

11

from an isolated protagonist. Osler's approach must be placed somehow within the enumerative category, stemming from a deep love of books.

At McGill University, the evidence of Osler's interest in books is everywhere. Osler learned to treasure books and to read them and know them in his family home, and he retained and nourished this feeling throughout his life. But it was also the man whom the book represented that interested Osler. His practice of being led from a consideration of the book to a consideration of the author characterized Osler's approach to history and to bibliography. Years later, in his discussion of Harvey's *De Motu Cordis* and *De Generatione*, the approach is mature and complete. History, and its usefulness to us, wrote Osler, "is directly proportionate to the completeness of our study of the individuals" who are the players in the rolls of history.[6]

By 1901, though, when Osler said, in Boston, that "books have been my delight these thirty years,"[7] his appreciation of books had broadened greatly from its beginnings. Books were now much more than vessels containing the magic of a name and words, or the mere repositories of knowledge. The beauty of books, the lure of variant printings and limited editions, the heady joys of collecting, all had been fully felt. And books about books had become important also.

In this address, Osler remarked on "the unique opportunities of the Surgeon-General's library." He saw that these opportunities were amplified through the *Index-Catalogue*—"one of the most stupendous bibliographical works ever undertaken . . . in it is furnished to the world a universal medical bibliography from the earliest times."[8] Osler's association with this library began early in his career and was by no means one-sided. As early as 1881 he invited Robert Fletcher to choose, from a list of books held in duplicate by McGill University, any that were needed in Washington; they would be " . . . a very slight return for the many handsome and valuable volumes received from the Surgeon-General's office."[9]

Osler worked even more directly in other areas that are bibliographical or impinge on bibliography; perhaps the most important of these relates to the founding of the Association of Medical Librarians. Osler is generally recognized as one of the three founders of this group, now the Medical Library Association.[10] He created or helped found a remarkable number of organizations, many of which exist today. He could identify genuine needs, sense who might successfully fill these needs, and support the early days of an organization with his name, his presence, his pen, and his pocket-book. The Association of Medical Librarians benefited in all these ways.[11]

Especially important to our purpose was Osler's election to the presidency of the Association in 1901, because it required a presidential address. In this address, entitled "Some Aspects of American Medical Bibliography," Osler gave a clear view of his approach to bibliography. He emphasized that he was "only a dabbler."[12] Is this an appropriate term, or was Osler being modest?

The address was vintage Osler, with all the Oslerian characteristics: frequent quotations from literature, classical and modern; generous mention by name of many who must have been in his audience; a style that is direct and clear; a practical message (". . . medical bibliography is worthy of a closer study than it has received heretofore in this country"[13]); and information that would both interest and instruct his audience.

What did Osler consider bibliography to be, in 1902? Well aware that "strictly speaking, bibliography means the science of everything relating to the book itself, and has nothing to do with its contents,"[14] he documented this definition by quoting Ferguson's *Some Aspects of Bibliography*. He identified three aspects of medical bibliography: " . . . the book itself, the book as a literary record, i.e., its contents, and the book in relation to the author."[15] The strict definition includes only the first of these three aspects. But to Osler there was a broader sense of the word "bibliography," and it is to this broad definition that he devotes his address.

The first section, on bibliography proper, occupies the least space in the published article; nor is that space much devoted to bibliography in the narrow sense. Osler wrote that typography in American medical imprints has little interest. Beyond that, he recommended collecting the early American periodicals and dilated enthusiastically on the value of the *Index-Catalogue* of the Surgeon-General's library. (As valuable as this research tool is, few today would second Osler's suggestion that authors might omit reference lists to their papers and simply refer to the *Index-Catalogue*.) In discussing books and their contents, Osler recorded his nominations of "certain treasures in American bibliography" which all should have on their shelves[16]—among others, John Morgan's *Discourse*,[17] John Jones's *Plain, Concise, Practical, Remarks on the Treatment of Wounds and Fractures*,[18] and Samuel Bard's *Angina Suffocativa*.[19] Finally, Osler discussed what he may have found the most congenial portion of his text: books and their

13

authors. He discussed " . . . writings which have a value to us from our interest in the author."[20] He believed that "there are men of noble life and high character, every scrap of whose writings should be precious to us. . . ."[21] (Did he suspect, by 1902, that he would be one of this company?) Oliver Wendell Holmes, S. Weir Mitchell, James Jackson, Daniel Drake—these and others earn Osler's accolade.

His interest in biography as history is well known. If his address on bibliography ends by drifting into history, we should not thereby be blinded to his contribution.

The Oxford Years

I have outlined some of Osler's bibliographical pursuits while he was in North America. In this phase of his career Osler could not be considered a bibliographer, but when he became Regius Professor at Oxford, in 1905, he began a productive fourteen years of work, much of which concerned bibliography. How did this happen?

Our attention must be directed to the Bibliographical Society. This society began with a paper delivered by W.A. Copinger to the Library Association, in 1891.[22] Copinger called for the creation of a bibliographical society, the inaugural meeting of which was held on July 15, 1892. Arrangements were made to publish annual *Transactions* (a policy that continued till 1920, when the Society took over *The Library*, which continues as the Society's official journal). Its first secretary was T.B. Reed, who was soon forced to resign because of ill health; he was succeeded by A.W. Pollard, the first of the great British bibliographers with whom Osler was associated directly. It was Pollard who created the concept of illustrated monographs as a medium for communication by the Society, and it was in this format that Osler's *Incunabula Medica* ultimately was published.[23]

Osler became a candidate-member of the Bibliographical Society in 1906.[24] When elected, Osler had been at Oxford for less than a year; his advent within the Society was seen accurately as a happy portent. Pollard recalled Osler's first attendance vividly: "A meeting had begun when the entrance of a stranger with an attractively mobile face, alert figure, and notably light tread caused a whispered secretarial inquiry as to who he was. The answer came that it was Professor Osler, and the secretary had an instinctive conviction that his coming meant much for the Society."[25]

Osler's impact, however, was not felt immediately. His first paper was not delivered until late in 1909, when he discussed "The Library of Robert Burton." Published originally in synopsis only,[26] the full text appeared posthumously in 1927.[27] Burton and his great *Anatomy of Melancholy* are such a pair as would inevitably transfix Osler's attention. The book he labelled unequivocally as "a medical treatise, the greatest indeed written by a layman."[28] He also identified the reason for its importance and its success: others who had written on the subject, Osler said, gained their knowledge from books, whereas Burton's came directly from "melancholizing."[29]

Osler noted that Burton was not a copious annotator; he remarked on the presence of such a few annotations in the books, adding the observation, "all of which have been looked over." But who had looked them over? The context, of course, allows no conclusion except that Osler had looked over all the books, but one marvels that Osler could manage to "look over" 1054 books, in the midst of his multifarious duties, hobbies and demands.

Studying these books enabled Osler to announce that "with but few exceptions the sources of the Burton river are easily traced, and they drain the whole territory of literature, ancient and modern, sacred and profane."[30] Osler was delighted with the sweep of Burton and the breadth of his reading, and especially with Burton's sympathetic observations on the foibles of "the motley procession of humanity."[31]

Osler gave his paper on Burton's library in 1909. The delivery of a "successful"[32] paper was customarily followed by the offer of a nomination to the Council, an offer that Osler accepted. Elected in 1910, he became a vice-president the following year. The prime candidate for the presidency was Abbot Gasquet, but because he took on increasing responsibilities as head of the Commission on the Vulgate at Rome, in 1913 Osler became president.[33]

He was elected to a second term in 1914. This term overlapped the beginning of the First World War, and, because the Council decided to make no changes during the war, Osler remained president for 7 years, the longest period in the history of the Bibliographical Society. As its historian has said, the Society "was doubly fortunate having Sir William Osler for President."[34] His enthusiasm, organizational ability, and capacity to stimulate others to extra efforts were all called into service. Cushing referred to "the usual obligations to the Bibliographical Society,"[35] and Pollard suggested that the Society survived "mainly . . . because its quiet meetings once a month during the winter were extraordinarily restful,"[36] mentioning Osler's continual labours in behalf of the Society. Thus Osler sponsored fourteen members and his name brought many others; much more important than the resultant external prosperity was the real inspiration he provided:

> His own zest and enthusiasm were infectious, and he was unfailing in the sympathy with which he cheered on those who were doing the spade-work for which it was impossible that he himself should find time. More than this: he worked out for himself a really noble conception of bibliography.[37]

In this instance Pollard referred not to the *Bibliotheca Osleriana* but to *Incunabula Medica*, a study of the earliest printed medical books, developed as Osler's presidential address to the Bibliographical Society in 1914. Throughout the war Osler tried to continue the detailed work needed on the actual bibliography that was to be published, along with the address, to make an esthetic bibliographic whole. He even authorized what Pollard termed "hopeful allusions" to it in the Society's annual reports. But the demands on Osler's time exceeded even his remarkable capacity and he made little progress. In 1918, Victor Scholderer, of the British Museum, was asked to coordinate the materials collected. Osler died before the work could be completed, and thus never saw the bibliography in its final form, as published by Oxford University Press in 1923.

The main essay was Osler's work, based on his 1914 presidential address. What does this address tell us about his bibliographic opinions and knowledge in 1914? His purpose was "to indicate the influence which the introduction of printing had upon medicine, to get, if possible, a mental picture of professors and practice at the time from the characters of books they thought it worth while to have printed."[38] No desiccated pedantry is evident here. Rather, and it is a recurrent theme, one notes the effort to show what long-dead persons thought and believed and felt.

The period that Osler studied covered 13 years, 1467-1480. After describing the medical therapy of the time succinctly, Osler then discussed current therapy, especially bleeding. Evidently he planned to include bleeding-calendars in the bibliography, but they were deleted, apparently because they had been thoroughly described by other workers.

The last half of the essay describes many of the books cited in Scholderer's bibliography. One excerpt gives the flavour of his commentary:

> A striking figure in the literature of the period is Peter of Abano, a little town near Padua, who shares with Arnold of Villanova the medical honours of the thirteenth century. A peripatetic professor teaching in Paris, Padua, and Bologna, he was known as 'Vir magnae sed audacis et temerariae doctrinae.' He has the honour to be one of the wise men for whom Naudé, by way of apology, wrote the *History of Magic*. He was several times accused of heresy, and it is said that he escaped condemnation only by his death. His books were prohibited, and a bundle of straw representing him was burned at Padua.[39]

Osler concluded his discussion of what he found a somewhat arid period in history by adjuring the sympathetic student to "look beyond the printed page to find in the lives of these men the spirit of helpfulness which gives to the profession of medicine its value to humanity."[40]

So the theme recurs. From books to men; from men to ideals and humanity. Osler's love of humankind was legendary. That he was able to transfer that love to his own modest studies in a traditionally dry area such as bibliography is, perhaps, a tribute to his humanism. On the other hand, bibliography is practised by bibliographers, and bibliographers are people, so Osler had to hand the raw materials he needed to find human values in bibliography as elsewhere.

British Bibliography

In Osler's day, Britain was the centre of the bibliographic world, or at least of the English-speaking portion of that world. No wonder Osler labelled his presidency of the Bibliographical Society "a very embarrassing honour."[41] The names resound in the ear of every bibliographer: A.W. Pollard, R.B. McKerrow, Sir Walter W. Greg, Falconer Madan, Cardinal F.A. Gasquet, Sir John Y.W. MacAlister, and Charles Sayle. Inevitably, one speculates on Osler's influence on these men.

First, though, a word about one precursor, James Atkinson, author of *Medical Bibliography. A and B* (1834). With him, Osler shared a commonality that may explain Osler's warm feelings about Atkinson and his book. It is a curious, droll and irreverent work, of only occasional bibliographic value. Atkinson's sense of humour is indicated by the fact that his book is not "unfinished," as one might suspect by observing that he treats only authors whose names begin with the letters A and B; that is all he intended to do. He cares not a whit what you think of him or his books, though his request for forgiveness is disarming:

> I pray you, gentlest of all gentle readers, to forgive me; and if there unfortunately be a magazine of fulminating powder in the criticising cell of your os petrosum, don't use a percussion lock or hair trigger; don't let it burst suddenly upon me; for I am of a nervous, quiet, and peaceable, though ridiculous nature; and far advanced in life. And you will have no credit in killing so harmless a creature.[42]

Osler's affection for Atkinson is intriguing, for there are superficial similarities between the bibliographical activities of the two men. Each, a physician, came to medical bibliography as a hobby; each approached his self-appointed task idiosyncratically; and each brought literary skill and an obvious affection for the form and substance of books to his bibliography. Moreover, the two men were soul-mates in that they shared a respect for the man behind the book.

With regard to the bibliographers of Osler's day, Pollard, Madan, MacAlister, and Sayle were, perhaps, especially close to Osler. Pollard,[43] an Oxford man, was associated with the British Museum from 1883 until his retirement in the 1930's. His association with Osler was close through Pollard's long-time labours as secretary of the Bibliographical Society and as a coeditor (with MacAlister) of *The Library*. Among his many scholarly achievements he is best known for numerous and important Shakespearian publications. His relationship with Osler is clear fom a note by Pollard cited by Cushing:

> Many of us will remember Sir William most vividly as the president of the Colophon Club, composed of London members of the Bibliographical Society who dine together two or three times in a session and entertain readers of papers, especially any who come from a distance . . . under Osler's chairmanship the Colophon dinners formed an extraordinarily pleasant climax to the Society's meetings. He was always in high spirits, always ready with some graceful compliment to the read-

ers of papers, and full of friendliness and good stories. No dinners were held during the war but he called for one in January 1919 and outdid himself in his efforts to make it a success, incidentally insisting on providing champagne on the patently false pretext that it was the Secretary's birthday! Many of those at this dinner never saw him again, but they could hardly have a brighter memory of him.[44]

Madan was successively, during Osler's time at Oxford, Sub-librarian at the Bodleian until 1912 and then Bodley's Librarian; he succeeded Osler as president of the Bibliographical Society. Because Osler, as Regius Professor at Oxford, was an *ex officio* Curator of the Bodleian Library, he saw much of Madan. In an obituary notice devoted largely to Osler's "firm and constant" friendship to the Bodleian, Madan also commented that "of his passion for the history and literature of Medicine, for old and interesting books in general, and for the bibliography of them, hardly enough" has been said.[45]

MacAlister was founding editor of *The Library*, in 1892, and long-time secretary of the Library Association and, latterly, secretary and editor for the Royal Society of Medicine. Osler's contacts with MacAlister were frequent, at least partly because MacAlister's activities encompassed both bibliographic and medical areas much trodden by Osler.

Sayle was, among other things, a poet and the librarian of Cambridge University. His most important contact with Osler came because of that post and he may be mentioned in conjunction with the *Bibliotheca Osleriana*. Sayle's writings cover a remarkable spectrum,[46] including drama, poetry, biographical notices, library brochures, and bibliography.

Among later bibliographers, Geoffrey Keynes stands out. Osler and Keynes became acquainted, in 1909, through a shared affection for the writings of Sir Thomas Browne.[47] Keynes's bibliography of Browne's writings was only the beginning of what continues to be a most distinguished bibliographic career for Keynes. Fulton claimed that Keynes invented the form now widely recognized as "bio-bibliography," a claim that Keynes says he himself never made,[48] and in response to my question, he stated that the plan of his bibliography was entirely his own.[49] Keynes outlined his bibliographic beliefs as follows:

I see no cause for shame in the admission that the bibliographical impulse was aroused by admiration for the work of these great artists, by interest in their lives and personalities, and by the desire to know more, of every aspect of the subjects that was to be found in the current books available in the shops and libraries. All this amounts to hero-worship, which might be foolish if directed to trivial and unworthy objects, but is not to be condemned when it finds heroes that *are* heroes and swans that will not turn out to be literary geese.[50]

How Osler would have nodded his head and applauded!

Not all that Osler touched in bibliography turned to gold. One project that had a strong bibliographical flavour did not come to fruition. Nonetheless, the idea was an intriguing one that may provide a further insight into his aspirations and dreams. The idea concerned a College of the Book.

It seems that Osler first recorded his proposal for a College of the Book in 1907; at any rate, Cushing quoted from an unpublished manuscript that dates from about that time. In such a college, he wrote:

> . . . men could learn everything relating to the Book, from the preparation of manuscript & the whole mystery of authorship, to the art of binding; everything from the manufacture of paper to the type with which the book is printed; everything relating to the press & to the mart; everything about the history of printing from Gutenberg to Hoe; everything about the precursors of the printed book: the papyrus, the rolls, the parchment & the vellum, even about the old writing on the burnt bricks of Nineveh; everything about the care of books, the Library lore, how to stack & store books; how to catalogue, how to distribute them; how to make them vital living units in a community; everything that the student should know about the use of books, his skilled tools in the building of his mind.[51]

Among the departments proposed was a School of Bibliography. The idea proceeded no further, though Osler did write to the President of Johns Hopkins University to request his comments and to inquire whether he thought that Carnegie funds could be obtained to finance the College.[52] There the matter seems to have rested until 1917 when, speaking in Aberystwyth, Wales, he proposed the establishment of a library school. This was a much more modest suggestion—indeed, by no means innovative—but he did emphasize again the need to teach "every aspect of bibliography."[53]

So far as I know, no College of the Book exists today, but the idea has not disappeared. It helped to inspire MacAlister to write about "The Osler Library" in 1919,[54] and in 1966, Thomas Keys appealed again for the establishment of "The College of the Medical Book."[55]

MacAlister wrote his fantasy for the volumes prepared as a surprise for Osler on his seventieth birthday. Claiming to have dreamed the event, MacAlister looks ahead to 1939 when Osler, a vigorous ninety-year-old, supervises from afar a futuristic library. No book ever leaves the building. No formal system of classification is followed, books being shelved "chronologically and according to size."[56] Printing presses, bindery, and similar departments are located within sound-proof areas. All of this is presented with evident reliance on Osler's opinions as discussed with MacAlister, or perhaps as mild parodies of these opinions. The result is a pleasant essay that probably has been read seldom since 1919.

Keys's effort is much more an offspring of Osler's hopes. Perhaps appropriately, Keys's address was the George Dock Lecture on the History of Medicine for 1966, for Dock was a student under Osler at the University of Pennsylvania. Keys quotes at length from Osler and proceeds to his own blueprint, a highly detailed one in which he not only proposes specific course but also identifies those who should teach. Will this particular Oslerian dream ever come true? It is a noble scheme.

"Not in 'Osler' "

Even more noble is the library Osler collected, and its catalogue. LeFanu has termed the *Bibliotheca Osleriana* "a monumental contribution to medical bibliography."[57] The book constitutes probably Osler's most enduring work in this area. He described his work in his introduction to the *Bibliotheca Osleriana* entitled "The Collecting of a Library."[58]

Although Osler had been collecting books for decades, it was at Oxford that he had both the opportunity and the income[59] to add substantially to his library. Moreover, it was during the Oxford years that Osler began to plan his idiosyncratic scheme of classification for his books: the Bibliotheca Prima, Secunda, Litteraria, Historica, Biographica, and Bibliographica, plus Incunabula and Manuscripts. Cushing has suggested how the idea for the plan of the catalogue developed:

it must have taken form while he was browsing in the Pepys Library in 1914. . . . Mr. Charles Sayle of the Cambridge University Library, of whom he saw much at this time, became interested in the project, and they had many a subsequent exchange of visits in Oxford and Cambridge, during the course of which the plan, of a 'Bibliotheca Prima,' 'Bibliotheca Secunda,' and so on, came to be crystallized.[60]

By 1916 Osler could write Sayle that the Prima grows "in mind and in shelves."[61] Throughout these last years, Osler would pick Sayle's "Bibliothecal brain"[62] again and again.[63]

So even during the disasters in France and Flanders, bibliographic work could go forward. It did not, however, go quickly or smoothly, so that, after Osler's death in 1919, his literary executors faced a prodigious task. Much deserves to be said of the four men who took on this task. Whether Osler planned it this way we do not know, but it seems appropriate in the light of his career that two of these men were Canadians, one an American, and one British. The American, Leonard Mackall, "that quaint and erudite wizard,"[64] remained largely a long-distance consultant but the others, W.W. Francis, R.H. Hill, and Archibald Malloch, were intimately involved.

Hill believed that the catalogue, the *Bibliotheca Osleriana*, was "the largest piece of bibliographical work connected with Osler's name."[65] While Osler himself left the work largely as an idea and an outline—he had intended to write entries on many of the books, and general introductions to the major sections of the catalogue—time decreed otherwise. It was left to Francis, Hill and Malloch to do what needed to be done, in the way that they believed Osler would have wished it completed.

The catalogue, an annotated enumerative bibliography, has proved its value since it was published in 1929. It is, as Lloyd G. Stevenson has said,[66] a catalogue to be read, which distinguishes it from most other works of similar purpose. Although it is not as readable as Atkinson's bibliography, the *Bibliotheca Osleriana* contains annotations that are instructive and sometimes entertaining.

Two examples must suffice. Commenting on *The Guardian Angel*, a novel by Oliver Wendell Holmes, Osler wrote that

The doctor in American fiction is strong only in New England, where he has reached a position difficult to match elsewhere. At the Shattuck Lecture, 1893, of the Massachusetts Medical Society—while the President was anointing the orator—looking over the 1200 men in the big

Mechanics' Hall, I received a definite impression that never before had I seen so large a collection of doctors with faces indicating breeding and pasture.[67]

And discussing Mrs. Gaskell's *Wives and Daughters*, he says:

Mr. Gibson has the true ring, and we follow him and that dear Molly in his wide range of practice—'to lonely cottages on the borders of great commons, to farm houses at the end of narrow country lanes that led to nowhere else.' There is a good account of the apprenticeship system . . . and the master's prescription for calf-love is delightful. The original is said to be Peter Holland of Knutsford, Cheshire, the father of the well-known physician Sir Henry Holland. Clare, Mr. Gibson's second wife, is a warning![68]

The *Bibliotheca Osleriana* draws the reader on from one fascination to another. Certainly it is one of Osler's floats to posterity, and a major achievement of his head and heart.

Conclusion

In Britain, Osler's influence on bibliography was minimal. The direction of British bibliography was set by others, particularly a few dedicated professionals. To their specialized labours Osler was a self-confessed outsider, but he was acquainted with all these men and had close friendships with several. It was through his personality and character, which reflected his particular approach, that Osler made his contributions to bibliography.

One of these contributions was an analogue of his contributions in many fields—his ability to inspire others to perform first-rate work. The *Bibliotheca Osleriana* was conceived by Osler but it assumed its splendid form through the work of three dedicated and talented librarian-bibliographers. *Incunabula Medica* was conceived by Osler to fill a gap in scholarship, but the bibliographical detail work was done not by him but by others, and the final product was published several years after his death.

Osler's work in bibliography illustrates one of his great gifts, the ability to identify problems, to identify problem-solvers, and to bring them together productively in a high proportion of instances. His skill touched large numbers of his contemporaries and helps to explain the affection they continued to feel toward him, long after his death.

Is there a moral to this story? As the Duchess said (in *Alice's Adventures in Wonderland*), "Everything's got a moral if only you can find it."

In my eyes, the moral is that one can make a contribution in almost any field by applying oneself with dedication and enthusiasm. Specialists are necessary but not sufficient for the work of the world. Setting aside internal medicine, in which he *was* a specialist, Osler accomplished much in a variety of fields in which he was very much an amateur, yet one who was interested in seeking and searching, and one who could by the great strength of his personality and humanity inspire others to important achievements.

To some people, bibliography is indeed a "dry, dusty, tedious, accursed, hateful"[69] endeavour, just as Atkinson described it. But it was not so to Osler. Nor did Osler ever make bibliography seem dry or dusty to anyone who reads him. He knew about "the impenetrable medium of a dense and dolorous cloud of bibliography,"[70] but that, most certainly, was never Osler's style.

The research for this chapter was supported by grants from the Hannah Institute for the History of Medicine, Toronto, and from the John P. McGovern Foundation, Houston.

Notes

1. F.T. B[owers], "Bibliography," *Encyclopaedia Britannica*. 1968 ed.
2. W.W. Greg, "Bibliography — A Retrospect," in *The Bibliographical Society 1892-1942: Studies in Retrospect* (London: The Bibliographical Society, 1945), pp. 23-24.
3. Greg, p. 24.
4. B[owers], pp. 588-9.
5. B[owers], p. 590.
6. William Osler, *The Growth of Truth as Illustrated in the Discovery of the Circulation of the Blood* (London: Henry Frowde, 1906), p. 28.
7. William Osler, "Books and Men," *Boston Medical and Surgical Journal*, 144(1901), 60-61.
8. William Osler, "Some Aspects of American Medical Bibliography," *Bulletin of Association of Medical Librarians*, 1(1902), 19-32.
9. Thomas E. Keys, "Sir William Osler and the Medical Library," *Bulletin of the Medical Library Association*, 49(1961), 28.
10. Jack D. Key, "The Medical Library Association Commemorative Medal, 1898-1975," *Bulletin of the Medical Library Association*, 64(1976), 45-47.
11. Keys, "Osler and the Medical Library," p. 128.
12. Osler, "American Medical Bibliography," p. 19.
13. Osler, "American Medical Bibliography," p. 20.

14. Osler, "American Medical Bibliography," p. 21.
15. Osler, "American Medical Bibliography," pp. 20-21.
16. Osler, "American Medical Bibliography," pp. 25-26.
17. John Morgan, *A Discourse upon the Institution of Medical Schools in America* (Philadelphia, 1765).
18. John Jones, *Plain, Concise, Practical Remarks on the Treatment of Wounds and Fractures; to Which is Added an Appendix on Camp and Military Hospitals* (Philadelphia, 1776).
19. Samuel Bard, *An Enquiry into the Nature, Cause and Cure, of the Angina Suffocativa, or Sore Throat Distemper, as it is Commonly Called by the Inhabitants of this City and Colony* (New York, 1771).
20. Osler, "American Medical Bibliography," p. 28.
21. Osler, "American Medical Bibliography," p. 28.
22. The information in this section derives substantially from F.C. Francis, "The Bibliographical Society: A Sketch of the First Fifty Years," in *The Bibliographical Society 1892-1942: Studies in Retrospect* (London: The Bibliographical Society, 1945), pp. 1-22.
23. William Osler, *Incunabula Medica: A Study of the Earliest Printed Medical Books, 1467-1480* (Oxford: Oxford University Press, 1923).
24. A.W. P[ollard], Preface, *Incunabula Medica*, by William Osler, p.v.
25. P[ollard], Preface, p. vi.
26. "November Meeting. Summary," *Transactions of the Bibliographical Society*, 9(1912), 4-7.
27. William Osler, "The Library of Robert Burton," *Oxford Bibliographical Society Proceedings and Papers*, 1, pt. 3(1927), 182-190.
28. Osler, "Library of Robert Burton," p. 183.
29. Osler, "Library of Robert Burton," p. 183.
30. Osler, "Library of Robert Burton," p. 186.
31. Osler, "Library of Robert Burton," p. 190.
32. P[ollard], Preface, p. vi.
33. P[ollard], Preface, p. vi.
34. Francis, "Bibliographical Society," p. 16.
35. Harvey Cushing, *The Life of Sir William Osler* (Oxford: The Clarendon Press, 1925), vol. II, p. 584.
36. P[ollard], Preface, p. vii.
37. P[ollard], Preface, p. viii.
38. Osler, *Incunabula Medica*, p. 3.
39. Osler, *Incunabula Medica*, p. 23.
40. Osler, *Incunabula Medica*, p. 31.
41. Cushing, *Osler*, vol. II, p. 344.
42. James Atkinson, *Medical Bibliography. A. and B.* (London: John Churchill, 1834), p. iii.
43. Walter W. Greg, "Alfred William Pollard," *DNB* (1941-1950).
44. Cushing, *Osler*, vol. II, p. 632.

45. F. M[adan], "The Late Sir William Osler, Baronet, M.D., F.R.S., &c.," *Bodleian Quarterly Record*, 2(1920), 298-9.
46. "The Writings of Charles Sayle," *Library*, 6 (1921-6), 82-89.
47. Geoffrey Keynes, "The Oslerian Tradition," *British Medical Journal*, 4(7 December 1968), 599.
48. Letter received from Geoffrey Keynes, 14 February 1979.
49. Letter received from G. Keynes, 14 February 1979.
50. Geoffrey Keynes, *Bibliotheca Bibliographici* (London: The Trianon Press, 1964), p. xi.
51. Cushing, *Osler*, vol. II, p. 81.
52. Cushing, *Osler*, vol. II, p. 81-2.
53. William Osler, "The Science of Librarianship," *Bulletin of the Medical Library Association*, 7(1918), 70-74.
54. J.Y.W. MacAlister, "The Osler Library," in *Contributions to Medical and Biological Research: Dedicated to Sir William Osler* (New York: Paul B. Hoeber, 1919), vol. I, pp. 111-121.
55. Thomas E. Keys, "The College of the Medical Book," *Bulletin of the Los Angeles County Medical Association*, 96(1 December 1966), 16, 24-25, 31; (15 December 1966), 23, 26-28.
56. MacAlister, "Osler Library," p. 117.
57. W.R. LeFanu, "The Bibliotheca Osleriana After 26 Years," in *W.W. Francis: Tributes from His Friends on the Occasion of the Thirty-Fifth Anniversary of McGill University* (Montreal: The Osler Society, 1956), p. 49.
58. William Osler, "The Collecting of a Library," *Bibliotheca Osleriana: A Catalogue of Books Illustrating the History of Medicine and Science, Collected, Arranged, and Annotated by Sir William Osler, Bt. and Bequeathed to McGill University* (Oxford: Clarendon Press, 1929; rpt. Montreal: McGill-Queen's University Press, 1969) pp. xxi-xxxii.
59. George Harrell, "Osler Practice," *Bulletin of the History of Medicine*, 47(1973), 651.
60. Cushing, *Osler*, vol. II, p. 417.
61. Cushing, *Osler*, vol. II, p. 531.
62. Cushing, *Osler*, vol. II, p. 571.
63. The mutual affinity of Osler and Sayle may be explained partially by noting that the latter edited editions of Sir Thomas Browne (*Bibliotheca Osleriana* no. 4526), wrote an essay about him (B.O. no. 4560), and published an anthology of writings about the ages of man (B.O. no. 5421) in which he included some of Osler's "Fixed Period" address (Cushing, *Osler*, vol. II, p. 547).
64. Mackall's role remains somewhat of a mystery, to me at least. Hill (*W.W. Francis: Tributes*, pp. 36-47) mentions his generous donations of expensive volumes, his remarkable knowledge of books, and his careful reading of

proofs. Cushing quotes from 9 letters Osler sent to Mackall, all relating to shared interests in books.

65. R.W. Hill, *W.W. Francis: Tributes*, p. 40.
66. Lloyd G. Stevenson, "Prologue," in *Bibliotheca Osleriana* (1969), p. xiii.
67. Osler, *Bibliotheca Osleriana*, p. 446.
68. Osler, *Bibliotheca Osleriana*, p. 439.
69. Atkinson, *Medical Bibliography*, p. 365.
70. Atkinson, *Medical Bibliography*, p. 365.

Medico-Historical Research in Medieval and Renaissance Manuscripts

Richard J. Durling

Only recently has medical history emerged as a distinct discipline. That it has at last acquired academic status and recognition is due not least to the example and enthusiasm of Sir William Osler. A leader of his profession, he showed, both in his writings and in the magnificent library of printed books and manuscripts he built up, a lively and informed interest in the medical past. It is appropriate in this symposium to concentrate on manuscripts and their potential contribution to our knowledge of medieval and Renaissance medicine.

Printed Catalogues of Manuscripts

Interest in the medical past seems to have developed slowly. Not until the mid-nineteenth century did librarians and historians actively seek out medieval and Renaissance manuscripts. In part this reflects professional historians' concentration on the seven liberal arts. If they touched on *scientific* subjects, they studied the quadrivium—that is, arithmetic, geometry, astronomy and music.[1] Another, more prosaic factor is that up to the 1850s it was difficult for students to gain access to medical manuscripts. Many of the great libraries had not been adequately catalogued, though the desirability and need for such access had occurred to such pioneers of sixteenth-century medical bibliography as Pascal Lecocq[2], Israel Spach[3] and Johann Georg Schenck[4], who included manuscripts in their lists of printed books. Printed catalogues were rare: only one catalogue of manuscripts and printed books was published in the 16th century—a catalogue by P. Bertius of the Leiden University library, which appeared in Leiden in 1595.[5] But interest grew in the seventeenth century: in Professor P.O. Kristeller's indispensable catalogue of catalogues, seventeen inventories are listed for this period.[6] Of one of these works, E. Bernardus' catalogue of English and Irish manuscripts published in Oxford in 1697, Kristeller remarks that it is "still indispensable, especially for some of the Cathedral Libraries."[7]

The Enlightenment led to renewed activity. A host of libraries were inventoried by such distinguished figures as A.M. Bandini, B. Montfaucon, Z.C. von Uffenbach and Humphrey Wanley. The total number of published catalogues in the eighteenth century exceeded 100, though only two were devoted solely to medical manuscripts. In 1746-47, J.C.V. Möhsen described the medical manuscripts in the Royal Library in Berlin[8], and in 1785 Johann Daniel Metzger listed those in the Royal Library in

Königsberg (now Kaliningrad)[9]—a veritable drop in the ocean! In the nineteenth century enterprising societies and academies were founded to survey manuscript holdings. Great work was done with the support of governmental bodies, as in France and Italy. The larger libraries, such as the Austrian National Library[10], the Bodleian Library in Oxford[11] and the British Library[12], sensibly compiled *summary* catalogues of their holdings. By modern standards these may be considered unsatisfactory but at least they supply essential information.

What is the situation today? In 1948, in the preface to the first edition of his *Latin Manuscript Books before 1600*, Kristeller could write that cataloguing of the manuscript collections had been completed in France, and had proceeded well in Great Britain, Belgium and a few other countries; large gaps existed for Spain, Italy and Germany.[13] Similarly, four years later, Kristeller observed that cataloguing was nearly completed for France and the United States, and was well advanced for Great Britain, Belgium, Holland, and Switzerland, though there were still gaps for Spain, Sweden, Austria, and Italy, and, unfortunately, for Germany, where so many collections had been destroyed or dislocated during the Second World War.[14] In the two decades since then, much has been achieved as a search through *Scriptorium*[15] and the supplements to Kristeller by G. Dogaer[16] and Ch. Lohr[17] show. Particularly in Germany a whole host of superbly organized catalogues has been produced by workers inspired by directives issuing from a special subcommittee of the Deutsche Forschungs- gemeinschaft (DFG). These directives were published in 1973 as the *Richtlinien Handschriftenkatalogisierung*.[18] In Austria, which had been backward, teams of workers are tackling the provincial and religious lib- raries under the supervision of Dr. Otto Mazal of the Austrian National Library; they have adapted the guidelines of the DFG.[19] Important cata- logues are appearing in Italy and Spain. A project is also under way to in- ventory the Latin manuscripts of the Soviet Union; this, it is hoped, will be followed by access to the catalogued material. Finally, in Poland, scholars have *inter alia* catalogued some of the holdings of the famous Biblioteka Jagellionśka and other libraries.

Locating Medical Manuscripts

Before I turn to catalogues of medical manuscripts themselves, I must mention one important innovation. At the instigation of the Comité international de Paléographie[20], a series of catalogues of *dated* and (usually) localized manuscripts in France, Belgium, the Netherlands, Austria, Italy and Sweden is being prepared.[21] This will facilitate the study of script to 1600; one will be able to work from manuscripts whose date and place are known to those undated and not localized.

With respect to medical manuscripts, our task is rendered considerably lighter by the recent publication of S.A. Jayawardene's checklist.[22] Printed in *Annals of Science* for 1978, this lists published catalogues of Western scientific manuscripts before 1600 and includes medicine (pp. 161-168). Although one cannot mention all of the 118 items enumerated by Jayawardene, some must be noted. Three are surveys of national and international scope. One cannot bypass A. Beccaria's detailed descriptions of some 145 pre-Salernitan manuscripts from the ninth to the eleventh century scattered all over Europe;[23] it gives us for the first time some insight into what was a very dark period. The scientific content is not great; mostly pseudepigrapha, lists of unlucky days, treatises on bloodletting and uroscopy, for example, are listed. The material, however, should be sifted and edited. Similar material was inventoried by the late doyen of French medical historians, Ernest Wickersheimer, whose catalogue of 118 manuscripts is limited to France of the early Middle Ages.[24] Wickersheimer occasionally duplicated Beccaria but tended to give more detail and edited selected portions of the texts. A third contribution is that of Guy Beaujouan, who recently carefully listed the medieval medical manuscripts of Spain.[25] This contains some genuine discoveries.

Among the catalogues of individual libraries, one must, of course, mention (taking a side-glance at the *Bibliotheca Osleriana* with its 162 manuscripts) the late Sam Moorat's catalogue of the Wellcome Institute of Medicine's rich holdings of manuscripts.[26] One must mention warmly also Dr. Dorothy Schullian's catalogue of the National Library of Medicine's manuscript collection, which, though small, is select.[27] A collection even smaller and, until recently, barely known or cited in the literature, is that in the Murhard Library, Kassel. This contains 21 medieval manuscripts and a few Renaissance items, excellently catalogued by Hartmut Broszinski.[28] Of ancient authors, Hippocrates is represented by his *Aphorisms*[29] and *Prognostics*[30] and Galen, by his *De Rigore*[31], *De Inaequali Intemperie*[32] and *Methodus Medendi*, books 7-14.[33] The *De Inaequali Intemperie* is accompanied by a marginal commentary; *both* were completed in Montpellier in 1336. Of Arabic authors, Kassel has a fine parchment Avicenna—his

33

influential *Canon*, book 1 only[34]—Abulcasis' *Liber Servitoris*[35], and the younger Serapion's *Liber Aggregatus de Medicinis Simplicibus*.[36] Of Salernitan authors, Kassel has Archimatthaeus' *Practica*[37], the mysterious treatise on female complaints known as *Trotula*[38], and the first Salernitan anatomical demonstration, the so-called *Anatomia Cophonis*.[39] Medieval *western* authors include Bernard of Gordon and his *Lilium Medicinae*[40], Gilles de Corbeil, who wrote *Carmen de Urinis*[41], and Gerard de Solo, author of the commentary on the ninth book of al-Razi's *Almansor*.[42] All these items and many more are meticulously described, with full codicological detail. In the case of paper manuscripts, care is taken to identify all watermarks with the aid of the standard repertoires.[43] Broszinski's catalogue could serve as a model for similar ventures.

Perhaps the most important recent contribution to manuscript studies is the *Catalogue of Incipits of Mediaeval Scientific Writings*, compiled by the late Professor Lynn Thorndike and Professor Pearl Kibre.[44] This lists thousands of texts in European and trans-Atlantic libraries. Their 23,000 incipits aid one to identify anonymous works. Note should also be taken of such projects as that of the cataloguing of medical manuscripts on microfilm at the National Library of Medicine, a programme begun in 1965. An extensive list of desiderata was drawn up largely on the basis of Thorndike and Kibre and Hermann Diels[45] (the latter includes Latin translations of Greek medical writings). The European libraries contacted cooperated magnificently, and by 1968 71 libraries between them had supplied 582 manuscripts on film.[46] Where possible, the entire codex, not just fragments or portions, was microfilmed. All manuscripts were then catalogued summarily, giving author, incipits, explicits, colophons, shelf-marks, and references where appropriate to Thorndike and Kibre or Diels, or both. The resultant card-files are available to visitors to the National Library of Medicine, and there is now a duplicate copy at the Institute for the History of Medicine in Kiel. The NLM is, alas, not empowered to make further copies of these microfilms for purposes of inter-library loan or outright purchase. The films must be consulted *in situ*.

There remains one important reference work that Jayawardene overlooked. This is Kristeller's two-volume *Iter Italicum*, published in 1963 and 1967, which spreads its net sufficiently wide to include no less than 1,174 manuscripts of interest to the medical historian.[47] Particularly important for the history of diagnosis and treatment are the sixty-one manuscripts containing *consilia* (advice for the patient). Modern critical editions of these are a major desideratum. Kristeller plans to publish shortly accounts of his manuscript searches outside Italy. I am sure he has reaped a rich harvest.

Deciphering Medical Manuscripts

So far we have concentrated on *finding* manuscripts: we come now to the problem of *deciphering* them. A well-written introduction to the subject is Professor James J. John's "Latin Palaeography" in the volume edited by James W. Powell, entitled *Medieval Studies: An Introduction.*[48] John divides the history of Latin script in the Middle Ages into three periods— early medieval or pre-Caroline, Caroline, and Gothic. He begins with the preceding Roman scripts: the square capital, the rustic capital, the uncial and half-uncial and the Roman cursives. Then, turning to pre-Caroline scripts, he successively deals with insular scripts (so-called because of their origin in Ireland or continued use in the British Isles), the visigothic minuscule, the Beneventan minuscule, and Merovingian scripts, the last of which can be difficult to read. He then discusses Caroline script, which lasted for more than four centuries, and finally he surveys the Gothic scripts. Small facsimiles of each script are provided.

Since most of the medical manuscripts we are likely to encounter belong to the later Middle Ages, it might be advisable to consult also the facsimiles and transcriptions provided by S. Harrison Thomson in his *Latin Bookhands of the Later Middle Ages, 1100-1500.*[49] Thomson has selected 132 manuscripts and has arranged them chronologically in reference to France, Germany, Italy, Britain and Iberia. Each manuscript is dated and localized. The transcriptions are preceded by paragraphs detailing the location and shelf-mark of the codex reproduced, its contents, its place of origin, and the characteristics of the script used, together with matters pertaining to orthography. I have found these last particularly helpful. Another useful selection, this time of medical manuscripts only, was made by Miriam Drabkin (*Bulletin of the History of Medicine*, 71 (1942), 409-436). There she reproduces excellent examples of scripts ranging from seventh-century uncials to fifteenth-century Gothic cursives. Brief notes describe the script and the abbreviations used. This brings us to the chief difficulty experienced by beginners: abbreviations. Indispensable guides here are A. Cappelli's *Dizionario di Abbreviature latine ed italiane* and Auguste Pelzer's *Abréviations latines médievales.*[50]

Editing Medical Manuscripts

After locating and deciphering manuscripts the next problem is editing them. The first question to consider is whether the text is contained in one manuscript only or in several. If only in one, one should probably attempt a diplomatic edition, preserving all the readings of the original and indicating the true readings in the critical apparatus. If the text is contained in several, it is necessary to collate each manuscript and to record its variants, using as the control (where available) a previously printed text. After each manuscript has been collated, readings must be compared and relationships established among them. One may contain all the errors (including omissions) of another as well as some of its own. The likelihood then is that it is a copy of the other and should therefore be eliminated. There is no point in retaining a completely derivative manuscript. One manuscript may share the errors of another but one may be right where the other is wrong and *vice versa*: neither, then, can be copied from the other and both must be retained to constitute their common ancestor. The object is to establish the lost ancestor of *all* known manuscripts, one so-called archetype. Classical scholars usually express the relationships of the manuscripts they retain for their editions in the form of a *stemma codicum*, or family-tree. It may not always be possible to draw up a *stemma* if there has been contamination, which occurs when, instead of copying one exemplar, a scribe compares different copies and records their readings in his own manuscript. One may express such contamination on the *stemma* in the form of dotted lines. The rules for stemmatics have been laid down in a difficult book by Paul Maas;[51] a distinctly more human guide is Professor M.L. West in his *Textual Criticism and Editorial Technique.*[52]

Classical scholars give to the first stage—the reconstruction of the most primitive state of the text recoverable from the manuscripts the term *recensio*. The next stage is termed *examinatio*, in which one asks whether this primitive state is authentic or not. If it is not, one must emend it (*emendatio*). For this last stage there are no rules, but the scholar must ask how the corruption arose. He must draw on his knowledge of the language and subject matter and of the thought processes of the author. He will not be asked in the case of medieval medical texts to perform prodigies—he need be no Bentley or A.E. Housman—but merely to display common sense. Too many editions of medieval medical texts—and I do not except the great Sudhoff—occasionally print nonsense.

This is a greatly oversimplified account, based on the excellent chapter on textual criticism in the guide of L.D. Reynolds and N.G. Wilson *Scribes and Scholars*.[53] There are some good remarks also in James Willis' *Latin Textual Criticism*[54], but the best introduction to the subject remains that of West, who gives useful hints for the would-be editor (61ff.)—yet, as he himself knows, no textbook made an editor. As in palaeography, we learn by doing; we also learn by imitating others. My own greatest debt is to the former editor of the *Aristoteles Latinus*, the distinguished Dr. L. Minio-Paluello, and his sometime collaborator, Professor Drossaart Lulofs, of Amsterdam. The editions for which both are responsible are exemplary, whether one considers the text or the *apparatus criticus* or not least, the Greek and Latin indices.

Lessons from Medical Manuscripts

What can medical manuscripts and archives teach us? They can teach us about the lives of physicians and their status in the community, their education, their salaries, their attitudes to their patients and their ailments, and their helplessness in the face of major disasters such as epidemics. Their treatments were mostly traditional and ineffective, a gigantic 'as if.' Consequently, too many general histories of medicine bypass the Middle Ages as offering little new or effective. Despite the efforts of De Renzi, Daremberg, Sudhoff, Wickersheimer and Sigerist—all of whom knew how to exploit manuscript materials—the general attitude of amused contempt prevails.

These scholars hardly got beyond assembling the evidence; they did not digest or interpret it. As a result, their researches are not really incorporated in the textbooks. Fielding Garrison summed it up with his usual precision, when, after pointing out that Sudhoff's bibliography ran to 700 items by the time he was 80, he remarked that "while much of this vast array of building material cannot, as yet, be made to function, it has undoubtedly determined the directives and objectives for the scientific investigation of medical history in the future."[55] An American scholar has recently used some of Sudhoff's materials to answer important questions concerning the medieval practitioner's attitudes toward his responsibilities in time of plague.[56] More work should be done on similar lines but with different perspectives.

The time has come to interpret the evidence already collected by previous generations. This does not preclude collecting still further material, editing texts, and writing commentaries, but there is a huge need for a synthesis on medieval medicine. We have for England an excellent account by Dr. Charles Talbot;[57] we have nothing similar for European medicine as a whole. Perhaps the time is not yet ripe. What Sigerist wrote in 1934 applies equally today: "The history of medieval medicine has not been written yet, and a satisfactory history of the period will require many more years of study in libraries and archives."[58]

Notes

1. Gerhard Baader, "Lo sviluppo del linguaggio medico nell'antichità e nel primo medioevo," *Atene e Roma*, N.S. 15(1970), 1-19.

2. Pascal (Paschalis Gallus) Lecocq, *Bibliotheca Medica* (1590; rpt. Geneva — Sampierdarena: Scuola Grafica Don Boscu, 1970). See his articles on Joannes Actuarius (p. 37), Avicenna (pp. 40-41) and Guy de Chauliac (pp. 116-117).

3. Israel Spach, *Nomenclator Scriptorum Medicorum* (Frankfurt am Main, 1591).

4. Johann Georg Schenck, *Biblia Iatrica* (Frankfurt am Main, 1609).

5. P. Bertius, *Nomenclator Autorum Omnium Quorum Libri vel Manuscripti, vel Typis Expressi Exstant* in *Bibliotheca Academiae Lugduno-Batavae* (Leiden, 1595). There is a copy in Leiden University Library. See P.O. Kristeller, *Latin Manuscript Books before 1600: A List of the Printed Catalogues and Unpublished Inventories of Extant Collections*, 3rd ed. (New York: Fordham University Press, 1965), pp. 134-135; hereafter referred to as Kr. According to G. Pollard and A. Ehrman, *The Distribution of Books by Catalogue from the Invention of Printing to A.D. 1800* (Cambridge: Printed for presentation to members of the Roxburghe Club, 1965), p. 343, the first library catalogue published was that of Cambridge, where in 1574 John Caius' *Historia Cantabrigiensis Academiae* appeared. This included a list of the MS holdings of the library. I owe my knowledge of this to Professor E.J. Kenney's excellent *The Classical Text: Aspects of Editing in the Age of the Printed Book*, Sather Classical Lectures, 44 (Berkeley and Los Angeles: University of California Press, 1974), pp. 86-87.

6. Paulus de Angelis, *Basilicae S. Mariae Maioris de Urbe . . . Descriptio et*

Delineatio (Rome, 1621), Kr., p. 214; E. Bernardus, *Catalogi Librorum Manuscriptorum Angliae et Hiberniae*, 2 vols. in 1 (Oxford, 1697), Kr., pp. 20-21; *Bibliotheca Norfolciana sive Catalogus Libb. Manuscriptorum et Impressorum . . . quos Henricus Dux Norfolciae etc. Regiae Societati Londinensi . . . donavit* (London, 1681), Kr., p. 143; *Catalogus Bibliothecae Lugduno-Batavae* (Leiden, 1640), Kr., p. 135; J. Feller, *Catalogus Codicum Manuscriptorum Bibliothecae Paulinae in Academia Lipsiensi* (Leipzig, 1686), Kr., p. 136; Thomas James, *Ecloga Oxonio-Cantabrigiensis*, 2 pts. in 1 (London, 1600), Kr., p. 39; Ph. Labbeus, *Nova Bibliotheca Manuscriptorum Librorum* (Paris, 1652-53), Kr., p. 40; P. Lambecius, *Commentariorum de Augustissima Bibliotheca Caesarea Vindobonensi*, 2 vols. in 4 (Vienna, 1665-69), Kr., p. 222; J. Mabillon and M. Germain, *Museum Italicum*, 2 vols. (Paris, 1687-89), Kr., p. 43; J.V. Marchesius, *Codicum mmss. Latinorum Vatic. Palatinae Bibliothecae Index* (1678), Kr., p. 212; A. Possevinus, *Apparatus Sacer*, 2nd ed., 2 vols. (Cologne, 1608), Kr., p. 53; *Petri Johannis Resenii Bibliotheca Regine Academiae Hafniensis donata* (Copenhagen, 1685), Kr., pp. 6 and 13; A. Sanderus, *Bibliotheca Belgica Manuscripta*, 2 vols. in 1 (Lille, 1641-44), Kr., p. 57; Th. Smith, *Catalogus Librorum Manuscriptorum Bibliothecae Cottonianae* (Oxford, 1696), Kr., p. 142; Th. Spizelius, *Bibliothecarum Illustrium Arcana Retecta* (Augsburg, 1668), Kr., p. 61; Jac. Phil. Tomasinus, *Bibliothecae Patavinae Manuscriptae Publicae et Privatae* (Udine, 1639), Kr., p. 171; *Idem, Bibliothecae Venetae Manuscriptae Publicae et Privatae* (Udine, 1650), Kr., p. 214; I. Atkins and N.R. Ker (eds.),*Catalogus Librorum Manuscriptorum Bibliothecae Wigorniensis, made in 1622-1623 by Patrick Young* (Cambridge: University Press, 1944), Kr., p. 225.

7. Kr., p. 21.
8. J.C.V. Möhsen, *Dissertatio Epistolica Prima (Secunda) de Manuscriptis Medicis quae Inter Codices Bibliothecae Regiae Berolinensis Servantur* (Berlin, 1746-47), Kr., p. 78.
9. Johann Daniel Metzger, *Medicinischer Briefwechsel* (1785). Contains: "Verzeichniss der medicinischen Handschriften auf der kgl. Bibliothek zu Königsberg," Kr., p. 126.
10. *Tabulae Codicum Manuscriptorum Praeter Graecos et Orientales in Bibliotheca Palatina Vindobonensi Asservatorum*, 11 vols. (Vienna, 1864-1912), Kr., p. 222. This is rich in medical material and well-indexed.
11. F. Madan, H.H.E. Craster and N. Denholm-Young, *A Summary Catalogue of Western Manuscripts in the Bodleian Library at Oxford*, 7 vols. (Oxford, 1895-1953), Kr., p. 169.
12. See Kr., p. 143 for details.
13. Kr., p. xvii.
14. Kr., p. xxiii.
15. Founded in 1947. See in particular its *Bulletin codicologique*.

16. G. Dogaer, "Quelques additions au répertoire de Kristeller," *Scriptorium*, 22 (1969), 84-86.

17. Charles H. Lohr, "Further additions to Kristeller's Repertorium," *Scriptorium*, 26 (1972), 343-348. See also G. Philippart, "Catalogues récents de manuscrits," *Analecta Bollandiana*, 88 (1970), 188-211.

18. (Bonn-Bad Godesberg: Deutsche Forschungsgemeinschaft, 1973). This is reviewed by A. Derolez in *Scriptorium*, 28 (1974), 299-300.

19. *Handschriftenbeschreibung*, Österreichische Akademie der Wissenschaften, Philosophisch-Historische Klasse Denkscriften, 122. Band, Veröffentlichungen der Kommission für Schrift-und Buchwesen des Mittelalters, Reihe II, Band 1, ed. Otto Mazal (Vienna: Verlag der Österreichischen Akademie der Wissenschaften, 1975), p. 132. This contains important contributions by Eva Irblich on the history of cataloguing in Austria (pp. 21ff.) and by Otto Mazal on the tasks, expectations, problems and limitations of the manuscript cataloguer (pp. 31-39). Mazal, after pointing out that the cataloguing of manuscripts goes back to the period of manuscripts themselves and that they were mostly the crudest of finding-lists, outlines the needs or demands of the modern researcher. He is only well-served if the main text is described exhaustively, and if further all notes, insertions, marginalia, glosses and fragments are registered; if the origin and dating of the script, the construction of the book, the artistic decoration, the binding, the history of the manuscript are all examined and the literature listed.

20. On the Comité and its programmes *see* Ch. Samaran in *Journal des savants* (1962), pp. 75-94; M.-C. Garand, in *Codices Manuscripti*, 1 (1975), 97-103.

21. See, for example, Ch. Samaran and R. Marichal, *Catalogue des manuscrits en écriture latine, portant des indications de date, de lieu ou de copiste*, 8 vols. (Paris: Centre national de la recherche scientifique, 1959-); G.I. Lieftinck, *Manuscrits datés conservés dans les Pays-Bas*, 2 vols. (Amsterdam: North-Holland, 1964); F. Masai and M. Wittek, *Manuscrits datés conservés en Belgique*, 2 vols. (Brussels, Ghent: E. Story-Scientia, 1968-1972); F. Unterkircher, *Die datierten Handschriften in der Österreichischen Nationalbibliothek*, 4 vols. (Vienna: Herman Bohlaus, 1969-1976); *Catalogo dei monoscritti in scrittura latina datati o databili per indicazione di anno, di luogo o di copista* (Torino: Bottega d'Erasmo, 1971-); M. Hedlund, *Katalog der datierten Handschriften in lateinischer Schrift vor 1600 in Schweden*, 2 vols. (Stockholm: Almqvist & Wiksell, 1977), and Beat Matthias von Scarpatetti, *Die Handschriften der Bibliotheken von Aarau, Appenzell und Basel*, Katalog der datier ten Handschriften in der Schweiz in lateinischer Schrift vom Anfang des Mittelalters bis 1550 (Zurich: Urs Graf Verlag, 1977).

22. S.A. Jayawardene, "Western Scientific Manuscripts Before 1600: A Checklist of Published Catalogues," *Annals of Science*, 35 (1978), 143-172.

23. Augusto Beccaria, *I codici di medicina del periodo Presalernitano, Secoli IX,*

X e XI (Roma, Edizioni di Storia e letteratura, 1956). See the reviews by Dorothy Schullian in *Journal of the History of Medicine*, 13 (1958), 106-109; Loren MacKinney in *Isis*, 49 (1958), 90-91; and Lynn Thorndike in *Speculum*, 32 (1957), 536-538.

24. Ernest Wickersheimer, *Les Manuscrits latins de medécine du haut Moyen Âge dans les bibliothèques de France*, Documents, études et répertoires publiés par l'Institut de Recherche et d'Histoire des Textes, 11 (Paris: Editions du Centre national de la recherche scientifique, 1966). This includes an impressive bibliography of Wickersheimer's publications, the majority on medieval medicine. For his work, see Marie-Thérèse d'Alverny, "L'OEuvre scientifique du docteur Ernest Wickersheimer," in *Humanisme actif: Mélanges d'art et de littérature offerts à Julien Cain* (Paris: Hermann, 1968), II, 299-307.

25. Guy Beaujouan, "Manuscrits Médicaux du Moyen Âge Conservés en Espagne," *Mélanges de la Casa de Velazquez*, 8 (1972), 161-221.

26. S.A.J. Moorat, *Catalogue of Western Manuscripts on Medicine and Science in the Wellcome Historical Medical Library*, 2 vols. (London: Wellcome Historical Medical Library, 1962-73). Vol. 1 reviewed by Curt F. Bühler in *Journal of the History of Medicine*, 18 (1963), 182-183.

27. Dorothy Schullian and F.E. Sommer, *Catalogue of Incunabula and Manuscripts in the Army Medical Library* now the National Library of Medicine, Bethesda, Md. (New York: Henry Schuman, 1950).

28. Hartmut Broszinski, *Manuscripta Medica*, Die Handschriften der Murhardschen Bibliothek der Stadt Kassel und Landesbibliothek (Wiesbaden: Harrassowitz, 1976).

29. Hippocrates *Aphorismi* 4° Ms. med. 8 ca. 1418, ff. 50^v-60^r; 8° 10, ca. 1336? ff. 23^v-44^v.

30. Hippocrates *Prognostics* 4^O8, ca. 1418, ff. 38^r-48^v.

31. Galen *De Rigore* 2^O8, s. xiv, ff. 1ra-4rb.

32. Here entitled *De Malitia Complexionis*, 8^O10, a. 1336, ff. 46^r-53^r.

33. Here entitled *De Ingenio Sanitatis*, 8^O10, a. 1332 (Goslar), ff. 53^r-105^r; the Arabic-Latin version is that of Gerard of Cremona.

34. Avicenna *Liber Canonis Primus* 2^O3, s. xiv, ff. 1ra-87vb.

35. Abulcasis *Liber Servitoris* 2^O4, s. xiv, ff. 1ra-16va.

36. Serapion *Liber Aggregatus* 2^O4, ca. 1300 (Italy), ff. 17ra-123vb.

37. Archimatthaeus *Practica* 2^O6, s. xiv, ff. 4va-8ra.

38. Trotula *De Passionibus Mulierum* 2^O7, ca. 1435, ff. 224ra-238rb.

39. *Anatomia Cophonis* (or *Anatomia Porci*) 2^O6, s. xiv, ff. 19va-20va.

40. Bernard of Gordon *Lilium Medicinae* 2^O7, ca. 1435, ff. 2^r-223rb.

41. Aegidius Corboliensis *Carmen de Urinis* 4^O8, ca. 1418, ff. 32^v-37^r; 8^O10, a, 1336, ff. 1^r-9^r.

42. Gerardus de Solo *Commentum Super Nona Particula Almansoris* 4^O16, s. xiv, ff. 55ra-124vb; 4^O21, ca. 1380, ff. 1^r-105^v.

43. Charles-Moise Briquet, *Les filigranes*, 2 éd., 4 vols. (Leipzig: K.W. Hierse-

mann, 1923); Vladimir A. Mošin and Seid M. Traljić, *Filigranes des XIIIe et XIVe ss*, 2 vols. (Zagreb: Académie Yougoslave des sciences et des beaux-arts, Institut d'histoire, 1957); Gerhard Piccard, *Die Kronenwasserzeichen* (Stuttgart: Kohlhammer, 1961); *Die Ochsenkopfwasserzeichen*, 3 vols. (Stuttgart: Kohlhammer, 1966); *Die Turmwasserzeichen* (Stuttgart: Kohl-hammer, 1970); Die Wasser-zeichenkartei Piccard im Hauptstaatsarchiv Stuttgart, Findbuch 1-3. The 1968 reprint of Briquet edited by Allan Stevenson brings the bibliography up to date.

44. Revised and augmented ed. (Cambridge, Mass.: Mediaeval Academy of America, 1963). Inevitably in a compilation of this scope errors were bound to occur. Some have been pointed out by the compilers themselves: Lynn Thorndike, "Additional Addenda et Corrigenda," *Speculum*, 40 (1965), 116-122; Pearl Kibre, "Further Addenda and Corrigenda," *Speculum*, 43 (1968), 78-114; see also Hubert Silvestre, "Les Incipits des oeuvres scienti-fiques latines du Moyen Âge," *Scriptorium*, 19 (1965), 273-278. In time to come, there will no doubt be a third edition. I hope the sponsors, the Mediaeval Academy of America, will consider the advisability of putting the entire work on computer. It can then be regularly updated by a team of scholars.

45. Hermann Diels, *Die Handschriften der antiken Ärzte*, (Berlin: Verlag der königlich Akademie der Wissenschaften, 1906). The First Nachtrag was published in 1908. This work also appeared in serial form in *Abhandlungen der königlich Preussischen Akademie der Wissenschaften, Philosophisch-historische Classe*, 1905-1907.

46. See *A Summary Checklist of Medical Manuscripts on Microfilm Held by the National Library of Medicine* (Bethesda, Md.: National Library of Medi-cine, 1968). The Wissenschaftliche Bibliothek Erfurt, the British Library, the Bayrische Staatsbibliothek München, the Bibliothèque Nationale Paris, and the Vatican Library proved especially cooperative.

47. See my review in the *Journal of the History of Medicine*, 24 (1969), 89-97.

48. (Syracuse, N.Y.: Syracuse University Press, 1976), pp. 1-68. A newly-revised article on palaeography by Professor Bernhard Bischoff will be ap-pearing in the next edition of *Deutsche Philologie im Aufriss*. In the mean-time see his article on the subject in *Dahlmann-Waitz Quellenkunde der Deutschen Geschichte*, ed. H. Hempel and H. Geuss, 10th ed. (Stuttgart: A. Hiersemann, 1969) I, Section 14.

49. (Cambridge: Cambridge University Press, 1969).

50. 6th ed. (Milano: Hoepli, 1967); 2nd ed. (Louvain: Publications Universi-taires, 1966).

51. *Textual Criticism*, tr. Barbara Flower (Oxford: Clarendon Press, 1958).

52. (Stuttgart: B.G. Teubner, 1973). See pp. 37-46 for advice on dealing with contamination.

53. 2 ed., rev. and enl. (Oxford: Clarendon Press, 1975), pp. 186-213.

54. James Alfred Willis, *Latin Textual Criticism*, Illinois Studies in Languages and Literature, 61 (Urbana, Ill.: University of Illinois Press, 1972).

55. "Karl Sudhoff as Editor and Bibliographer," *Bulletin of the Institute of the History of Medicine*, 2 (1934), 8.

56. Darrel W. Amundsen, "Medical Deontology and Pestilential Disease in the Late Middle Ages," *Journal of the History of Medicine*, 32 (1977), 403-421.

57. Charles H. Talbot, *Medicine in Medieval England* (London: Oldbourne, 1967).

58. Henry E. Sigerist, "Karl Sudhoff the Mediaevalist," *Bulletin of the Institute of the History of Medicine*, 2 (1934), 25.

Looking Forward
Into Historical
Medical Bibliography

Estelle Brodman

Osler's interest in books and historical and descriptive bibliography is too well known to require attention here, but it is pertinent to ask how historical medical bibliography has fared since Osler's day and how one might expect it to develop. In order to answer these questions it will be helpful to describe medical bibliography and medical bibliographers at the end of the nineteenth century, to enumerate the social conditions that affected them, to review the present state of the art, and then (placing firmly on my head the conical hat worn alike by idiot and seer) to peer into the future and suggest what medical bibliography might be like in the next half-century.

Medical Bibliography Before the First World War

As I look back and try to discern what life must have been like in civilized countries at the turn of the present century, what strikes me most is the feeling of hope at that time—in such contrast with our present gloom and pessimism, and our general feeling of frustration and inability to influence life about us. Actual living conditions were probably far worse than at present—long working hours, insufficient wages, poor housing, malnutrition, political graft, high infant mortality—but in general things were better than they had been, and technological, medical, and social advances beckoned to an even brighter future. The world, one could say, was getting better every day in every way.

In the field of bibliography, this belief in the possibility of better relations between peoples and nations, in the universality of science above nationalism, and in the new techniques for wide dissemination of information (such as the Mergenthaler Linotype machine and the rotary press, which made possible the cheap daily newspaper, and the underwater cable, allowing for an international telegraph service) led to the birth of several schemes for universal scientific bibliography. It is no accident that Paul Otlet's International Bibliographic Institute or the Universal Decimal Classification scheme were propounded around the turn of the century, and many librarians of my age can remember the unfiled cards from the Concilium Bibliographicum in Brussels that haunted our daily rounds—a universal bibliography founded with such hope when Victoria was still on the throne, and which limped along until after the First World War, killed as much by internecine strife as was Revere Osler in battle.

In the hope that medical sciences could improve the quality and duration of life, and in the further belief that all civilized countries were con-

47

tributing to that advance, physicians and scientists could and did work to make medical information from everywhere known to everyone. (I emphasize 'civilized' countries because few people are aware that the old *Index-Catalogue* systematically omitted most Australasian Journals, on Osler's comment in 1897 "that they contain little except records of hydatids and snake-bite."[1]) Simultaneously, scientists of all European nationalities were sending references to publications from their countries to the Royal Society in London for a joint publication, in a scheme, many of whose ideas are echoed in UNESCO's present UNISIST program.

Out of this shining hope for a universally cooperating world came the *International Catalogue of Scientific Papers*; Virchow's *Jahresbericht*; and the great bibliographers of medicine, John Shaw Billings and the *Index-Catalogue*, Neale and his selective *Medical Digest*, Pauly and his annotated *Bibliographie des sciences médicales*, Schmidt and his *Jahrbücher*; and also William Osler and the school of medical historians and bibliographers that has come down to our day. I need only refer to the direct succession from Osler to Cushing to Fulton to Sir Geoffrey Keynes, and the perhaps less direct but strongly Osler-influenced line of bibliographers, such as Janet Doe, Noel Poynter, or William Bean, to make my point.

But this breed of bibliographers is a dying one. Why is this so? Certainly it is not due to a dearth of bibliographies. There is hardly a subject— scientific, literary, educational, or humanistic—for which a list of more or less pertinent references has not been compiled and somehow published. What John Shaw Billings said in 1902 still holds true. "Many schemes for bibliographies, general, special, annotated, etc., have been suggested, and a few have been . . . tried. Each of these, from the universal bibliography to contain thirty millions of titles, to the bibliography of posters or of Podunk imprints, or of poems and essays condemned by their authors, has at least one admirer and advocate in the person who would like to have charge of the making of it; but when it comes to the question as to what has a commercial value there is great unanimity on the opinion that many of these bibliographies should be paid for . . . by government or by some philanthropic individual."[2] But these bibliographies are usually grab-bags of books and articles—"bibliography by the yard", it has been called. They contain everything the compiler could learn of on the subject, with the good, bad, and indifferent jumbled together; they are usually arranged impersonally by the alphabetical and accidental sequence of authors' names and they tend not to be annotated or described, summarized or compared.

What is lacking today is not bibliographies but evaluative bibliographers in the Oslerian-Cushing-Fulton-Keynes tradition. The scholar-collector who knows his subject so thoroughly that he can act as artist is rare at any time; but today he is generally too busy to give time to that slow process of learning, then presenting his knowledge to others, which is the *sine qua non* of fine bibliography. True bibliography requires the same art of selecting and highlighting used by the painter, which focuses attention on important areas and thus brings to our attention facets of the scene we would not otherwise have noticed. Tolstoy describes this in *War and Peace*, when he compares scientific history to the artist's depiction of the same event, and concludes that the artist presents the truer picture. Thus W.B. McDaniel II, reviewing Janet Doe's bibliography of Ambrose Paré in the 1930s, characterized it as "a strikingly fine work" because the author "vitalized her bibliography by discussing the subject of it in relation to his books and the books in relation to the time, place, and circumstances which brought them forth." He further wrote that her entries were full, leisurely and discursive, providing a history of the several texts in their transmission to readers and students throughout a period of nearly four centuries.[3] Much more recently a modern bibliographer, Katharine F. Pantzer, editor of Volume 2 of the revised *Short-Title Catalogue* (1976) was praised for her "delightful candor, which is unheard of in bibliographies [and which] comes from a thorough knowledge of the books as well as an understanding that this kind of wide-range bibliography is never finished. It recognizes that bibliographies are compiled through human decisions and that complete objectivity of analysis and presentation is a never-to-be-reached ideal . . ."[4] In such bibliographies complete objectivity is the abnegation of responsibility; it is like offering guests uncooked chickens and raw carrots, rather than a succulent dinner.

The Influence of Technological Developments on Bibliography

But I do not wish to seem to denigrate either the value of unevaluated lists or the effect of changes in bibliography caused by societal pressures and technological developments. One cannot end up with that delectable rabbit stew of Escoffier fame without first catching the rabbit; nor would a reasonable person eschew the advantages of modernity in favor of Miniver

Cheevy's longing for *le temps perdu*. Here is where enumerative bibliography comes in, as the underpinning for critical bibliography. It is the necessary, if not sufficient, requirement of the Oslerian-type bibliographer. And here is where the advances of the past half-century have been so startling and so exciting.

Enumerative bibliography has as its aim the recording of all material in its field; and if to some it has the same soporific quality as the "begats" of the Bible or the catalog of ships of the *Iliad*, it still serves an equally important role with these classics in documenting data from which the artist-bibliographer can select what is to be highlighted.

This fact has been understood and appreciated by most bibliographers since at least the sixteenth century. Symphorien Champier, for example, in his *De Medicine Claris Scriptoribus* (1506), tried to bring together the medical literature of several countries with the special purpose of transmitting the new discoveries of Renaissance Italy to his French colleagues. Since his time and down to today the goal of enumerative bibliography has always been to diminish the effects of geography and language on the transmission of data and on its interpretation.

Just as people have always used the most efficient methods known to them to accomplish whatever goals they had in mind, so enumerative bibliographers in each generation have adapted the technical advances of their time to their tasks. Thus, when printing became widespread, the technologic advance brought in the detailed citation of edition, volume, and page, made possible—even mandatory—when all copies of a work were exactly the same. It also allowed the once-for-all reproduction through printing of the ensuing bibliography in much larger numbers than was possible in the old hand-copying commercial factories. This in turn brought down the price of an individual exemplar of the bibliography so that even a poor scholar could afford one. Having further enlarged the desire of the scholar for the works cited, this new technologic advance led to the growth of larger libraries, often supported by great patrons and governmental bodies, the only ones (then as now) who could afford their collection and upkeep.

As the scale of publication increased—Ploucquet lamented as early as 1808, "we are blinded by too much light . . . no day passes but someone throws another article upon this mountain of material"[5]—it became impossible for individual bibliographers to examine all the literature. A system of joint bibliography became necessary, of which the Royal Society's *Catalogue of Scientific Papers* and John Shaw Billings' *Index-Catalogue* are the outstanding examples up to Osler's time. Billings, indeed, even adapted to his bibliography the just-developing factory system of the time, in which jobs were standardized, broken up in parts, and distributed to a hierarchy of workers, each of whom did a single part only. (In a sense, of course, this is what all monumental and continuing bibliographies do even today.)

What caused the breakdown of this system was the same problem Ploucquet had been unable to solve: the technical advance of the printing press did not allow for the speedy addition of new material to the old. Ploucquet himself tried to solve it by publishing supplements, which at more or less lengthy intervals would be intercalated into the old lists and published again. Billings tried publishing a monthly index that could stand on its own (the *Index Medicus*) for newly appearing literature that might not be listed in the *Index-Catalogue* for fifteen to twenty years. And Melvil Dewey considered the card catalog as the answer to this problem, even though it restricted the use of the information to those who could come to the one catalog maintained by an institution.

This unsatisfactory state of affairs lasted until after the Second World War, when one of the technologic advances exploited for military purposes changed the situation. This was the digital computer, though it was not until the selenium chip replaced the vacuum tube for transmission of electrical impulses that the computer became a reasonable tool for bibliography. Later still came the printed circuit, which made possible today's mini-computers and microcomputers. No longer was it necessary to attempt, often unsuccessfully, to unite punched cards, card catalogs, and electronic printers.

Another interim solution to this problem was the joint use of punched cards, the automatic Listomatic Camera, and photoprinting to produce the *Current List of Medical Literature* in a design propounded by Seymour Taine, then its editor, and through development underwritten by the Council on Library Resources. It worked creakily and with difficulty, and lasted only until a truly computerized system could be established in the 1960s. Here the main protagonists were Taine, Frank B. Rogers, Director of the National Library of Medicine, and the staff of General Electric. In essence it is a system that was used to produce the *Index Medicus* and MEDLARS. It provided a speedy way of printing a general bibliography as well as a

51

method for producing subsets of this general bibliography, by combining various elements of the total in customized fashion. Thus, while the printed bibliography might list separately works on pneumonia, on untoward results of treatment with a particular antibiotic, and on the disease in humans under the age of five, MEDLARS could combine these topics by Boolean algebra and produce a single list of articles with all these topics in them.

What still had to be done, and what was dependent on the development of still newer technologic advances, was the presentation of this information to the inquirer in his own institution and at almost the instant of inquiry. For this an on-line reactive system between the inquirer and the computer was required. This led to MEDLINE (MEDLARS-On-Line) and a host of derivatives, such as CANCER-LINE, TOXLINE, and even HISTLINE for the history of medicine. Emboldened by the success of these, other indexing groups began similar systems. Commercial companies sprang up to provide access to these systems and to educate users in their use (or to raise demands for their middleman services, if one takes a cynical view of the situation), and networks of libraries were formed to act as brokers between the commercial vendors and the libraries using the services. Before anyone was aware of it a new industry was born. Some librarians, also, attempted to set up as specialists in the use of these data bases, while the whole field of clinical librarianship was based on the ability to obtain speedy access to newly published literature.

One other result of the introduction of on-line technological developments to bibliographic endeavors must be mentioned: the effect on cataloging. One job of the historian in any field is to examine evidence—evidence usually in the form of documents, as books or journals (though one must not underrate the importance of artifacts, of course). Locating these books and journals has always been difficult, made lighter perhaps by the bringing together in one place of the records of the holdings of many institutions. In addition to the *Short-Title Catalogue*, the *Gesamtkatalog der Wiegendrücke*, the National Union Catalog at the Library of Congress, the *Union List of Serials*, and the *Union Catalog of Medical Periodicals* (UCMP) are all examples of such joint documentation. All of these attempts, however, have suffered from the difficulty of keeping them up to date that Ploucquet and Billings encountered (even the *Union Catalog of Medical Periodicals*, which is published quarterly on microfiche); and some have required access to a unique card catalog record which may be in a remote city.

With the advent of the on-line computer system developed in the late 1960s and early 1970s, however, such new union catalogs as those in the Ohio College Library Center (OCLC) in Columbus, Ohio, and the Ballots system at Stanford University could be established. These can be a large part of the answer to the problem of speedy location of material needed by the bibliographer or other scholar. It is also possible, because of standardization of cataloging rules, for the bibliographer using these on-line systems to compare the title-page, names of editors and translators, publishers, and subjects of the book he has with those of books held in other institutions. Often, also, the original catalogers will have added notes to the formal portion of the catalog citation that will clarify obscure points the inquirer might have in *his* copy. And if all else fails he knows where to go to see the other copy himself. In the library of Washington University School of Medicine, for example, the cataloging of two large-scale rare book collections have been placed in the OCLC computer store and the catalog cards generated from it for our card catalog made available.

The Future

Exactly what the future will hold is impossible to say, but I think bibliography—both enumerative and critical bibliography—will continue to be important and will develop in line with the technologic state of the art of the day. For example, computerized typewriters will lead to storing, editing, re-editing, annotating, and changing of information directly onto a magnetic tape for reproduction in a variety of ways for wide distribution at a comparatively small cost. Long-line facsimile reproduction by telephone may sometime provide access to material too rare to subject to transportation from place to place or too fragile to allow most visitors to touch. There will undoubtedly be other advances. Printed biomedical indexes will wither away in favor of their on-line forms—for economic reasons—and on-line terminals will be united with home TV sets and be found in most laboratories and offices of the future paperless society. Whether this will occur in the next decade or before the end of this century is uncertain, but it is likely to come during the lifetime of young students of today.

But all these things are means to an end. They provide the bibliographer with the totality of information, with the externals. Still required will be the bibliographer following in the Oslerian tradition who must select from the total store, who must identify and study documents, and who must place them in relation to the milieu from which they emanated in such a way that they illuminate the subjects discussed. As in the past, what is needed is the artist-bibliographer, who is as important to the life of letters as the philosopher-king is to our civic life. Let us hope that both may flourish and grow.

Notes

1. F.H. Garrison in a memorandum (5 August 1929) quoted in Estelle Brodman, *The Development of Medical Bibliography* ([Baltimore]: Medical Library Association, 1954), pp. 115-16.
2. John Shaw Billings, "Some Library Problems of Tomorrow," *Library Journal*, 27 (1902), 1-9, reprinted in *Selected Papers of John Shaw Billings*, comp. Frank B. Rogers ([Baltimore]: Medical Library Association, 1965), pp. 249-262.
3. *Bulletin of the Medical Library Association*, 45 (1957), 282.
4. Paul S. Koda, "The Revised *Short-Title Catalogue* (STC); a Review Article," *Library Quarterly*, 48 (1978), 308.
5. Wilhelm Gottfried Ploucquet, *Literatura Medica Digesta* (1808-14) quoted in Brodman (note 1), p. 79.

Physical Bibliography
in the Twentieth Century

G. Thomas Tanselle

G. Thomas Tanselle

The fiftieth anniversary of the opening of the Osler Library provides a fitting occasion for a review of some of the twentieth-century developments in bibliography, for Osler was one of the illustrious examples of a collector who was also a bibliographer. His greatness as a scholarly collector is widely recognized, and if his service to the cause of bibliography is perhaps less well known, it is effectively symbolized by his seven years' presidency of the Bibliographical Society (1913-19). Those were the last seven years of his life, the years of the First World War, and the important years in bibliographical history just after the Bibliographical Society, in F.C. Francis's words, had "come of age," having reached its twenty-first birthday the year Osler became president.[1] The Society, according to Francis, was "doubly fortunate" to have Osler as president during the difficult wartime years, and his encouragement of and enthusiasm for matters bibliographical have been attested to by A.W. Pollard.[2] For years Osler had recognized the value of an integrated approach to all aspects of the study of books. When he delivered the inaugural address at the Summer School of Library Service at Aberystwyth in 1917, he set forth an idea he had started to develop in an unfinished paper of ten years earlier.[3] "I should like," he said, "to see added to the schools of at least one University in each division of the kingdom a *School of the Book*, in all its relations, historical, technical, and commercial—every aspect of bibliography, every detail of typography, every possible side of bibliopoly."[4] All these studies have advanced considerably since Osler spoke, but his call for an overview that ties them together is as timely as ever. When specialties develop, there is a tendency for workers in one area to lose touch with what is going on in another. But all bibliographical studies are complementary, and progress in our knowledge of the history of books can best be made through cooperation among those working on particular approaches or in particular fields.

I should like, therefore, to trace briefly certain movements in twentieth-century bibliography, in the hope that such a survey can help us to assess where we now stand and to think about our future prospects. The word "bibliography," as we all know, can mean many things, but I wish to focus on what is sometimes called, for want of a better term, "physical bibliography"—that is to say, the study of books as physical objects. The history of printing, publishing, and the book trade is obviously one branch of this study, and such history has often been based largely on documents external to the books themselves—documents such as printers' and publishers' business records, contracts, correspondence, and advertising. But what has been particularly characteristic of the twentieth century is the development of techniques for analyzing and recording the physical details present in the actual products of the printing and publishing process. These details, after all, must also be part of the raw material for more comprehensive histories; indeed, they constitute the primary evidence, for the details present in surviving artifacts must take precedence over reports about those artifacts in external documents. The branches of bibliography specifically concerned with these matters have come to be called analytical bibliography and descriptive bibliography. The analytical bibliographer develops techniques for examining pieces of printed matter with a view to deducing, from the physical evidence found within them, as much as possible about the history of their production; the descriptive bibliographer records in an orderly fashion the physical details present in particular editions, impressions, and issues in order to provide a standard description against which further copies can be compared. Clearly these pursuits are interrelated, for the identification and classification that accompany description must rest on analysis. However, analysis can serve ends other than description: the principal impetus to the development of analytical bibliography in the twentieth century has been the role it plays in the editing of texts. Thus the physical study of books has a bearing on the study of the intellectual content of books. In fact, changing perceptions of this relationship form one of the motifs of twentieth-century bibliographical history. One could think of the course of development of analytical and descriptive bibliography as a double movement: they have come more and more to be recognized as activities that produce results of interest in their own right, activities that are not merely ancillary to the study of literature; in the process they have become more intertwined and begun to make an even greater contribution to literary study. Furthermore, although scholars of literature have been the primary developers of twentieth-century analytical and descriptive bibliography, it should be clear that printed materials of all kinds—not only those considered to contain belles-lettres—are proper subjects for bibliographical investigation; it should be equally clear, but frequently is not, that such investigation is important for the study of printed materials in all fields.[5]

If analytical and descriptive bibliography can be thought of as products of the twentieth century, they nevertheless have behind them some nineteenth-century, and even eighteenth-century, antecedents. Michael

58

Maittaire's chronological treatment of incunabula in the early eighteenth century (*Annales typographici*, 1719-41) and Joseph Ames's *Typographical Antiquities* at mid-century (1749; revised by William Herbert, 1785-90) set the stage for G. W. F. Panzer's study (*Annales typographici*, 1793-1803), which arranged incunabula so that the output of individual printers was kept together under each year. These works reflect a gradual development of interest in books as physical artifacts, symbolized by the priority Panzer gives to arrangement by printer over arrangement by author or type of work. It was not until the third quarter of the nineteenth century, however, that this approach became truly analytic, in the hands of Henry Bradshaw, who believed that bibliographical study could be put on a scientific basis by pursuing what he called the "natural history method." Just as a natural scientist could classify a specimen of a previously unknown species in relation to other already classified specimens, so a bibliographer should be able to assign a piece of printed matter to its proper time, place, and printer by comparing its features with those of other examples the identity of which is already known. This kind of analysis requires an arrangement of entries by country, then by town, then by printer, and then by year, with the order of the countries, towns, and printers established by the date of the earliest imprint associated with each; it also requires close attention to typographic details and peculiarities. Bradshaw is thus with good reason regarded as the father of analytical bibliography, for his work suggests for the first time in a systematic and extended way some of the kinds of things that can be learned from a careful study of the physical evidence present in pieces of printed matter. His approach influenced many other scholars, both in Britain and on the continent, most notably Robert Proctor, whose *Index to the Early Printed Books in the British Museum . . . with Notes of Those in the Bodleian Library* (1898) is the first great monument of analytical bibliography. It would be hard to overestimate the importance of Bradshaw in bibliographical history. At the same time, one should recognize where analytical bibliography stood at the beginning of the twentieth century: it consisted principally of well-developed techniques for comparing letter-forms in the process of identifying printers of incunabula; little thought had been given to other techniques that might prove more appropriate for books of later periods or to the possibility that physical evidence might have a bearing on the study of the intellectual content of books.[6]

While Bradshaw and his followers were at work in the last quarter of the nineteenth century, another development was taking place that is also

significant for twentieth-century bibliography. In contrast to the undisci-
plined enthusiasm for book collecting represented by the writings of
Thomas Frognall Dibdin in the early part of the nineteenth century, there
began to appear in the 1870s an interest in the more systematic recording of
the first editions of particular authors, principally nineteenth-century authors. Various so-called bibliographies appeared, often the work of
Richard Herne Shepherd, C. P. Johnson, J. P. Anderson, and C. B. For-
man; but it was the bibliographies by T. J. Wise, extending well into the
new century, that came to symbolize the whole movement, just as his own
personal influence had affected the choice of authors most avidly collected.[7] Wise's later notoriety, resulting from certain other of his practices,
should not cause one to overlook his formative role in the early days of descriptive bibliography.[8] He directed attention to nineteenth-century books,
to the preservation of them in their original boards or cloth casings, and to
the importance of author-bibliographies as reference tools for collectors and
dealers. The conception of author-bibliography that he fostered, however,
was a quite limited one. He did not recognize the extent to which an accurate record requires the examination of multiple copies (he was inclined to
believe that his own copies set the standard), nor did he conceive of a
bibliography as more than a guide to the identification of first editions or
impressions. He did not, in other words, see individual books against the
background of book-production history nor think of collecting as an activity that required such knowledge.

As the twentieth century began, therefore, an unfortunate split existed in bibliographical work between studies aimed at scholars and those
aimed at collectors. The nature of the early publications in analytical bibliography and descriptive bibliography was readily taken to mean that
bibliographical analysis was important in the scholarly study of early
books, whereas author-bibliographies, especially of more recent books,
could satisfy the needs of collectors without getting involved in elaborate
analysis or in reporting details that seemed to be unnecessary for the inden-
tification of firsts. This notion that collectors are not scholars and that they
require different reference books from those for scholars has proved to be a
hard one to eradicate, and its effects are still being felt, nearly a century
later. If analytical and descriptive bibliography seemed in some respects to
be moving in different directions at the turn of the century, they were alike
in tending to concentrate on specific limited goals; recognition of the larger

purposes they served—the way in which they contributed to each other, to publishing history, to editorial work, and thus ultimately to literary criticism—had not yet been generally perceived. An important shift took place, however, in the early years of the new century, one that was not without problems of its own, because it resulted in some bibliographical activities being thought of not as ends in themselves but as preparation for literary study. Nevertheless, in the hands primarily of literary scholars, analytical and descriptive bibliography have flourished in the twentieth century. If it is now time to insist that they are independent pursuits relevant to all fields that utilize printed matter and not simply to "literature," the argument does not question the great benefits to bibliographical study that have occurred as a result of the turn that bibliographical history took just after the beginning of the century.

I

Three great scholars of English literature—R. B. McKerrow, A. W. Pollard, and W. W. Greg—are justly recognized as the founders of modern analytical bibliography.[9] All three were interested, among other things, in the English dramatic literature of the Renaissance, and all demonstrated, in the first decade and a half of the century, the way in which the scholarly editing of those dramatic texts depended on a knowledge of printing-house practice of the time and on a close examination of the physical features of multiple copies of the printed texts. It is not surprising that this material should have been the source for a new and seminal kind of bibliographical analysis: much of it was great literature, the product of a period of extraordinary richness and vitality in the development of the language; very few manuscripts from this period survive, forcing one to scrutinize the printed texts for evidence of what had been present in the manuscripts; the routines of printing were such that authors frequently did not have an opportunity to read proofs, and uncorrected type pages as well as corrected ones appeared in the published books; the state of orthography gave the compositors in the printing shop considerable latitude to alter spellings according to their preferences or the exigencies of spacing; and the routes by which dramatic texts could reach the printing house meant that some published versions had been printed from copy only tenuously related to the author's own manuscripts. These conditions taken together provided the ideal breeding ground for techniques designed to extract from printed books evidence for deciding at what points the texts printed in them conformed to their authors' intentions and at what points they did not. Whereas the incunabulists had examined physical evidence in order to elucidate printing history by identifying or dating particular items, the scholars of Elizabethan and Jacobean drama investigated physical evidence in order to learn about the reliability of the text contained on the printed pages. In the process they obviously learned much about printing history, but the significant fact is that their primary interest, unlike that of the incunabulists, was in literature, not examples of printing. Their work is the first sustained demonstration of an important truth: that an analysis of the physical evidence associated with a piece of printed matter plays an important role in understanding what is being said in the writing conveyed by that printed matter.

The foundations of this new study were laid in a series of landmark publications early in the century. McKerrow set the stage for future scholarly editions when in his edition of Nashe (1904-10) he adumbrated the significance of printing history for editing by noting variants discovered in the collation of multiple copies of a single edition. Then Greg, in two articles in 1908, used watermark and typographical evidence to demonstrate the false dating of the Pavier quartos of Shakespeare.[10] And Pollard the following year published a more comprehensive examination of the physical basis for Shakespeare's texts in *Shakespeare Folios and Quartos*, a book that was a turning point in Shakespeare studies by firmly establishing the distinction between the "good" and the "bad" quartos. The most influential work of all, however, was the long piece that McKerrow contributed to the Bibliographical Society's *Transactions* in 1913 with the significant title, "Notes on Bibliographical Evidence for Literary Students and Editors of English Works of the Sixteenth and Seventeenth Centuries."[11] These hundred pages were expanded in 1927 to the three hundred fifty of *An Introduction to Bibliography for Literary Students*, a book that remained the basic guide to the field for half a century. The titles of both editions make clear that the emphasis was on bibliography as a servant of literature, and the preface of the 1927 volume is explicit on the subject: the book "still retains," McKerrow says, "the original idea of a help-book for literary students. I wish there to be no misunderstanding about this. It is not a hand-book for students of printing or of general bibliography." Even

McKerrow, however, could be guilty of a superficial view of book collecting, for he goes on, "Still less is it intended for book-collectors. I have not concerned myself in the least with the rarity or beauty or commercial value of the products of the printing-press, but have kept before me throughout the problem of the relation of the printed book to the written word of the author" (p. vi). Despite the unfortunate support given here to the distorted position that there is a gap between book collecting and bibliographical scholarship, McKerrow's book was a great positive force: to some extent it was a history of printing practices, but this aspect of it was subordinated to an exposition of certain techniques for extracting from printed matter data relevant to textual concerns. One comes to understand, in reading his book, that bibliographical analysis not only will make possible sound editing but will ultimately rewrite printing history as well. The book suggests more directions for fruitful investigation than definite answers to questions: much of its appeal comes from the sense it conveys of the excitement of being on the threshold of a promising new field. It may have become dated in the information it sets forth, but it has remained a valuable introduction to generations of bibliographers for the general approach and frame of mind it represents.[12]

If the brilliance of this outburst of bibliographical activity was not matched by what followed in the period between the two world wars, those years nevertheless witnessed the continued development of certain analytical techniques applied to Renaissance drama. In particular, the idea that variations in spelling, in the formation of contractions, and in the treatment of speech prefixes, scene headings, and stage directions could serve to differentiate the sections of text set by different compositors was pursued by several scholars. The belief underlying compositor analysis, of course, is that if some of the characteristics of individual compositors can be identified, then it may be possible to postulate certain ways in which the copy from which a compositor was setting differed from what appears in print, and one may thus be taken a step nearer to the author's manuscript. Pollard wrote on this subject,[13] but the most prominent of the newer names during this period was that of E. E. Willoughby, whose 1932 book *The Printing of the First Folio Shakespeare* not only utilized spelling evidence but also foreshadowed future work in its analysis of the typographical evidence of headlines, rules, and the like to demonstrate the order of sheets through the press. Other books of these years which, while less analytical in themselves, helped record the factual foundation on which further analysis could be based were Percy Simpson's *Proofreading in the Sixteenth, Seventeenth, and Eighteenth Centuries* (1935) and R. W. Chapman's *Cancels* (1930). The Chapman book was one of an extraordinary series of books edited by Michael Sadleir, under the title of "Bibliographia" but with the more revealing subtitle "Studies in Book History and Book Structure." These books focused on post-Renaissance material and are but one manifestation of the important role Sadleir played in the development of the bibliography of more recent books. Publisher and collector himself, he was the leader of a circle of dealers, collectors, and bibliographers who were at this time altering the course of twentieth-century bibliography by demonstrating through their activities the connections between collecting and scholarship and by illustrating the importance of applying analytical techniques to nineteenth- and twentieth-century books. The most spectacular publication to emerge from this group was of course John Carter and Graham Pollard's *An Enquiry into the Nature of Certain Nineteenth Century Pamphlets* (1934), which not only exposed the T. J. Wise forgeries but in the process showed that the analysis of type and paper was important for recent books as well as for books of the Renaissance.[14]

Despite the significance of these books, the next real surge in bibliographical activity did not occur until the years following World War II. The directions to come were suggested just before the war and during its early years in work by Fredson Bowers and Charlton Hinman on running titles, by William H. Bond on half-sheet imposition, and by W. W. Greg on proofreading practices.[15] The material examined in these studies continued to be English books (principally those containing plays) of the sixteenth and early seventeenth centuries, and the promising lines of inquiry opened up in them began to be thoroughly explored in the post-war years, especially by Bowers and Hinman and other scholars influenced by them. Bowers's founding in 1948 of an annual volume, *Studies in Bibliography*, to be sponsored by the Bibliographical Society of the University of Virginia, was the single most important symbolic landmark. Bowers made Virginia a center for bibliographical studies, and the journal provided a public forum for the presentation of the new bibliographical analysis. This kind of work appeared in other journals as well, but *Studies in Bibliography* became particularly associated with the encouragement of new techniques of analysis. What was new was the sophistication with which physical evidence was examined, with the consequent discovery of additional typographical features that could be made to yield significant information. Spelling analysis continued to be used, but a characteristic of the new school was the more intensive study of typographical peculiarities. Thus pieces of type that were distinctively damaged could be recognized upon their reappearance, and a careful tabulation of the recurrences of recognizable types in a given book could provide information about the timing of the distribution of type from one forme and the composition of type for another forme.[16] Because of the presence of recognizable types and rules in running-titles, the repeated use of particular running-titles in skeleton-formes could be identified, providing a powerful tool for use in determining the orde of formes through the press.[17] Although articles engaging in this kind of analysis do not make easy reading—some would even call them unreadable—many of them are fascinating for their ingenuity in extracting a considerable amount of information from intractable, and at first sight unpromising, data. The most sustained instance of bibliographical analysis is Hinman's examination of the Shakespeare First Folio, based on the eighty copies in the Folger collection. By skillfully employing all these techniques of analysis, his great work of 1963, *The Printing and Proof-Reading of the First Folio of Shakespeare*, not only proposed a page-by-page account of the printing history of the Folio but also served as an encyclopedic summation of the method and a dramatic demonstration of what it could achieve.

Post-Renaissance books have been the subject of far less extensive bibliographical analysis, although the early volumes of *Studies in Bibliography* did include some of William B. Todd's articles on press figures and other aspects of eighteenth-century bibliography—articles illustrating how fruitful analytical techniques applied to eighteenth-century books could be and showing at the same time how those techniques would have to be adjusted to fit the different conditions of eighteenth-century printing and publishing.[18] A few years later a promising series of short papers by Oliver L. Steele appeared in *Studies in Bibliography* and elsewhere, taking up the analysis of format and of plate damage in nineteenth- and twentieth-century books.[19] The approach used by Steele has not thus far been pursued to a great extent; but in the last two decades a considerable amount of bibliographical analysis of post-Renaissance books has taken place in connection with certain comprehensive scholarly editions of individual authors,[20] and it is inevitable that more analysis of this kind will take place in the future. The work began on incunabula, moved to Renaissance books, and now has been applied to more recent books, with results that should have convinced even the most skeptical of the need to examine books of all periods, down to the present, in the same analytical spirit.

That there has in the last few years been something of a pause in the great outpouring of analytical articles which began in the late 1940s is perhaps due to a feeling on the part of some that such analysis has become overly sophisticated and ingenious, that it has become an intellectual puzzle with little connection to the real world. This feeling was given its most consequential expression in D. F. McKenzie's long essay of 1969— also in *Studies in Bibliography*—called "Printers of the Mind."[21] As his title implies, McKenzie was concerned about certain bibliographical discussions that postulate, for purposes of analysis, a greater regularity and efficiency in the printing process than were likely to have existed in actuality and then accept the results of the analysis as demonstrated facts. Undoubtedly some conclusions were too hastily and confidently drawn, and his questioning of the procedure was timely. But his criticisms do not undermine the validity of analytical bibliography as a field of endeavor, when practiced with due scholarly caution, and it would be a matter for regret if his remarks cause able investigators to turn to other fields. The primary evidence for learning about the printing of books must be what is found in the books themselves; surviving documents and business records relating to printing and publishing activities obviously provide valuable supplementary information, but it should be clearly recognized as supplementary, because it is external to the objects, the pieces of printed matter, under investigation. Difficulties in drawing conclusions from evidence exist in all fields that employ inductive investigation; in bibliography, a general framework for thinking about the validity of inductive generalizations has been provided by Fredson Bowers in his Lyell Lectures of 1959, published as *Bibliography and Textual Criticism* (1964). Working within those guidelines, bibliographers should be encouraged to continue the analytical examination of books of all periods; only through the groundwork of detail that this kind of investigation can provide will there ultimately be a significant increase in our historical knowledge of printing and publishing practices.

The way in which the course of development of a field periodically turns back upon itself, placing earlier work in a new perspective and drawing it into the current stream, can be illustrated by one further achievement of analytical bibliography: the application of modern techniques of analysis to incunabula, as in Irvine Masson's *The Mainz Psalters and Canon Missae 1457-1459* (1954) and, especially, Allan Stevenson's *The Problem of the Missale speciale* (1967). Whereas most analysis has focused on the inked type-impressions on the pages of books, Stevenson looked for the evidence that could be found in the paper on which books were printed. In a series of important articles in the early volumes of *Studies in Bibliography*, he established the field of the bibliographical analysis of paper; his work was parallel to the new analytical studies of printing being undertaken at the time, and he was able to add to the analytical bibliographer's repertory of techniques several relating to paper.[22] Although his discoveries were relevant to all pre-nineteenth-century books, his own most sustained inquiry was into a fifteenth-century book, the so-called Constance missal. His 1967 study thus marked a return to the material that engaged the earliest analytical bibliographers, but with a point of view developed through three-quarters of a century of further analysis, principally devoted to books of subsequent periods. The celebrated problem of the Constance missal, which extensive analysis of typographical evidence by the earlier incunabulists had not been able to solve, was handled brilliantly by Stevenson, with the use of the paper evidence. He explicitly placed his work in the context of the twentieth-century development of "a form of enquiry known as analytical bibliography" (p. 26), acknowledging that the principal attention of this field had been concentrated on Elizabethan books and that one of the few serious uses of evidence from paper occurred at the very beginning, in Greg's 1908 investigation of the Pavier quartos. What he did not go on to say was that his own work, inspired by decades of physical analysis that had as its ultimate goal the establishment of texts, was directed toward the same goal that the earlier incunabulists' work had been—that is, the identification of the place and date of printing of a particular item. Stevenson was not interested in the text of the Special Missal any more than his predecessors had been, but he found the approach to analysis used by those concerned with Elizabethan dramatic texts to be congenial, indeed essential, to his purpose.

His work is thus a convenient way of demonstrating what I am suggesting as one of the chief directions of twentieth-century bibliography: the development of techniques for learning about book production, at first motivated by a desire to learn about the texts printed in those books, can then be recognized to have a more direct interest to those whose central concern is the history of book production. Because of the way analytical bibliography has grown, it is too often thought of as subordinate to literary studies, when actually, of course, its results are of interest in their own right and can emerge from an examination of any book, whether the contents are "literary" or not. We know much more about the printing of Elizabethan books than we would have known at this point if a body of great dramatic literature had not appeared in them; but we do not know as much, even about the books with dramatic texts, as we would have known if still more books of the period, including those with texts of little interest, had been investigated. Analytical bibliography has prospered in the twentieth century as a servant of literature; but the more it is recognized as an independent pursuit—returning in one sense to its nineteenth-century origins—the more it can be of use to literary studies, and to studies of all other kinds of texts as well.

II

Something of the same kind of evolution can be seen in descriptive bibliography. Although the author bibliographies of the late nineteenth century do not compare from the point of view of scholarship with the work of the incunabulists of that period, what is similar in the early development of the two areas is the way in which the same group of men just after the turn of the century made major contributions to both, affecting the future direction of each field. Before Pollard, Greg, and McKerrow undertook to systematize the recording of physical details about books, author bibliography was largely identified with somewhat superficial listings for collectors of nineteenth-century writers. But when Pollard and Greg in 1906 published in the Bibliographical Society's *Transactions* an essay called "Some Points in Bibliographical Descriptions,"[23] their manner of approaching the subject made clear that descriptive bibliography was a form of historical scholarship and that there was a value in having certain details on record, whether or not those details were essential for identifying first editions. That the same men who were developing analytical bibliography in connection with the editing of literary texts were also concerned with descriptive bibliography helped to suggest the relationships between the two and to show that descriptive bibliographies were important tools for the serious study of an author's writing. Although the relevance of Pollard and Greg's work to the description of more recent books was not widely recognized for a long time, the standards of description developed for Renaissance books— like the techniques of analysis for which the same men were responsible— had an enormous influence on the future activity in the field as a whole.

A series of important discussions of description followed, establishing the tradition within which we still operate. Pollard in 1907 wrote on "The Objects and Methods of Bibliographical Collations and Descriptions";[24] McKerrow included an account of what had become the standard form for descriptions in his 1913 "Notes on Bibliographical Evidence" and his 1927 book; the Oxford Bibliographical Society in 1922 published a statement on "Standard Descriptions of Printed Books" by Falconer Madan, Gordon Duff, and Strickland Gibson;[25] and Greg authoritatively set forth the details of collation formulas in 1934.[26] By the time of the Second World War, then, a basic form of description had been worked out, including title-page transcriptions, formulaic registers of signatures showing the essential physical structure of the books, an accounting of the contents of all the pages, and paragraphs on various physical features; and certain prominent examples of careful scholarly description were available, including the early volumes of the *Catalogue of Books Printed in the XVth Century Now in the British Museum* (1908-   ) and of Greg's *A Bibliography of the English Printed Drama to the Restoration* (1939-59). In the immediate post-war years Bowers played as decisive a role in descriptive bibliography as in analytical bibliography by bringing out a comprehensive treatise, *Principles of Bibliographical Description* (1949).[27] What gave that book its great authority was its firm grounding in the work of the preceding decades and its carefully reasoned extensions of traditional practice. It built on what had gone before, offering a systematic codification of established conventions, but it also expressed a rationale of description, provided definitions of such terms of classification as *impression, issue,* and *state*, discussed the description of machine-printed, as well as hand-printed, books, and buttressed those discussions with a wealth of examples from all periods. The book was an act of creative summary, providing for its field a basic guide of a kind that does not yet exist for analytical bibliography. Since 1949 some further work on the rationale and standards of description has occurred, especially Allan Stevenson's long introduction to the second volume of the *Catalogue of Botanical Books in the Collection of Rachel McMasters Miller Hunt* (1961) and several essays by Bowers himself;[28] but the 1949 book still stands as the authority in the field.

Although the major part of Bowers's book deals with pre-nineteenth-century material, his section on nineteenth- and twentieth-century books opens with a perceptive analysis of the shortcomings of much of the bibliographical work devoted to this period and of the reasons for them. Because many so-called bibliographies of authors of this period have been produced by people untrained in scholarly methods and publishing history, many of those bibliographies, he says, are "still in the semi-enumerative stage masquerading as descriptive" (p. 361) and have "scarcely advanced beyond the ideals and dubious standards" of their "godfather," T. J. Wise (p. 364). Bowers was not the first to see the need for more scholarly standards in bibliographies of machine-produced books, and it is worth recalling once more the role of the Sadleir circle in fostering an enlightened and responsible approach to bibliographical work on nineteenth- and twentieth-century books. In 1924 Iolo A. Williams explicitly stated in his book *Seven XVIIIth Century Bibliographies* that he was recording more details than were necessary for identification because of their potential future usefulness, thus revealing his view of a descriptive bibliography as a storehouse of details reflecting printing and publishing practices. It was Sadleir himself, however, who provided the most eloquent statement of this view and the most forceful example of it in his *Trollope: A Bibliography* (1928). The subtitle, beginning "An Analysis of the History and Structure of the Works of Anthony Trollope," makes clear the orientation of the work, and the preface begins by emphasizing "the general as opposed to the particular element" in the usefulness of the book. Bibliography, he says, "can be made to illustrate, not only the evolution of book-building, but also the history of book-handling and the effect of a gradually perfected book-craft on the aims and achievements of authorship." He regarded his Trollope bibliography, then, as "not only a reference work for collectors of that particular author but also a commentary on the book and publishing crafts of mid-Victorian England," and he believed that readers interested in other Victorian authors "will find in this compilation facts and deductions applicable to books with which Trollope had no concern whatsoever" (p. ix). Sadleir saw, as few others at the time did, that author bibliography is history, the history of the publication of an author's works and, as such, a part of the larger history of publishing in the period. This point of view was far from the one that prevailed among bibliographers of nineteenth-century books; it implied some acquaintance with the way books are put together and with how to analyze them, and it suggested that the goal was an understanding of the publishing conditions that determined the form of a given author's books. It held, in short, that author bibliography involved the pursuit of knowledge, not simply the listing of points for the identification of particular editions—though it is hard to see how the latter activity could in fact be performed satisfactorily in the absence of the former. Sadleir continued to be a leading spokesman for this enlightened position and made it the theme of his account of the bibliography of nineteenth-century books in the Bibliographical Society's *Studies in Retrospect* (1945), where he says that an emphasis on publishing history is "the principal quality which distinguishes to-day's practice from that of yesterday" (p. 154).

Despite the strength of this statement and of the one in Bowers's *Principles* four years later, it would be too much to say that this point of view has informed most author bibliographies since mid-century. Although one might have expected an increase in sophistication and thoroughness as a result of Bowers's book, the truth is that the proportion of praiseworthy bibliographies in the years since 1950 seems scarcely higher than the proportion that characterized earlier years. We can all think of certain prominent examples from before as well as after 1950: such series as Geoffrey Keynes's (1914-   ), the Soho Series (1951-   ), and the four volumes published by the Indiana Historical Society (1944-52), and such individual bibliographies as Henrietta C. Bartlett and A. W. Pollard's *Shakespeare* (1916, 1939), Frederick A. Pottle's *Boswell* (1929), William M. Sale's *Richardson* (1936), Hugh Macdonald's *Dryden* (1939), Jane Norton's *Gibbon* (1940), Allen T. Hazen's *Walpole* (1948), and Norma Russell's *Cowper* (1963), as well as those devoted to particular presses, such as Allen Hazen and J. P. Kirby's on the Strawberry Hill Press (1942, 1973), Philip Gaskell's on Baskerville (1959) and the Foulis Press (1964), D. F. McKenzie's on the Cambridge University Press (1966), and C. William Miller's on Benjamin Franklin (1974). The mid-century point does mark a kind of division in that before then there were very few serious bibliographies of more recent authors, but beginning at that time more of them started to appear: one thinks not only of certain of the Keynes, Soho, and Indiana volumes but also of Donald Gallup's *T. S. Eliot* (1952,

1969), Richard L. Purdy's *Hardy* (1954), and B. C. Bloomfield and Edward Mendelson's *Auden* (1964, 1972). All these titles are only examples, of course, and all in one way or another leave something to be desired, but most people would agree that they do stand out above the general level of bibliographies, before or after 1950—nor principally because of their adherence to particular formal conventions but because of the serious scholarly approach they exhibit.[29]

If the quantity of worthy bibliographies has not appreciably risen in the past quarter-century, what does characterize some of them, and distinguish them from their predecessors, is the use of new techniques and an approach to evidence influenced by the development of analytical bibliography. For example, in 1957 Matthew J. Bruccoli, in his *Notes on the Cabell Collections at the University of Virginia*, was able to identify separate impressions of some Cabell books by means of textual variation and plate damage discovered through collation on a Hinman Collator and by means of the measurement of inner margins ("gutters"). Similarly, Warner Barnes, in his bibliography of Elizabeth Barrett Browning (1967), reports for the first time many variations among copies, turned up through the use of the Hinman Collator. William B. Todd's bibliography of Burke (Soho, 1964) regularly records all press figures, not just those that serve to identify impressions, recognizing the function of a bibliography to provide a detailed historical record. Both James L. W. West III, in his bibliography of William Styron (1977), and Joel Myerson, in his bibliography of Margaret Fuller (1978), make use of recently suggested techniques for supplementing Bowers's *Principles* in the description of publishers' bindings, and West also employs the results of recent work on the description of type and paper. Myerson's bibliography is a volume in the Pittsburgh Series in Bibliography (1972-   ), which is noteworthy for its generally high standards and its hospitality to newer techniques. Although there is variation in practice among the volumes of this series, certain of them (such as Jennifer Atkinson's *O'Neill* of 1974) are notable for recognizing that later impressions (not just firsts) and material reprinted in anthologies (not just first appearances) are important elements in an author's publishing history and deserve to be recorded. West's bibliography of Styron merits recognition for another feature besides use of new descriptive techniques: its collation of texts as a routine part of description and its unusually thorough recording of textual variants discovered in the process. West collates not only copies of individual editions—in order to locate possible variants distinguishing states or impressions—but also copies of different editions—so that he is able to say how the text of a piece differs between its magazine appearance and its first book printing, for instance, or between two different editions in book form. This kind of information is unquestionably an important part of publication history, but descriptive bibliographers of the past have generally felt that they could not undertake the textual collation of all the books they describe. West's bibliography, in this as in other respects, represents the most recent bibliographical thinking, and it stands as an instructive example of how an excellent bibliography of today differs from excellent bibliographies of previous decades.

All these features in recent bibliographies help to move descriptive bibliography in the same direction that Sadleir pointed fifty years ago. And even now such bibliographies are exceptions. It still comes as a revelation to some people that the descriptive bibliography of an author can be regarded as a history or as a form of biography, that it is not simply a formulaic listing but instead is a study of the physical embodiments of an author's words, sorting out the relationships among those various embodiments, recording their physical characteristics, and setting forth (on the basis of this internal evidence and any available external evidence) the circumstances surrounding their printing and publication. That bibliographies of modern books are beginning—just beginning—to give more attention to textual collation is a reflection of the fact that the most intensive physical examination of nineteenth- and twentieth-century books has occurred in connection with comprehensive editions that have been under way during the past two decades. Although one may lament that the major nineteenth-century American authors have not yet been supplied with modern bibliographies, one can in fact find much of the information that would go into such bibliographies in the editorial matter appended to the multi-volume editions issued under the auspices of the Center for Editions of American Authors (CEAA) and its successor, the Center for Scholarly Editions. One cannot undertake a scholarly edition without having available the information that a scholarly bibliography would provide; and of course the attention to textual matters entailed by the research for an edition uncovers bibliographical facts. Just as the work on Elizabethan dramatic texts earlier served as a stimulus for the development of the descriptive bibliography of books of that period, so it remained for a large undertaking like the CEAA to concentrate enough attention on nineteenth-century texts so that the books containing them began to be approached with the historical focus Sadleir had called for. The rarity with which bibliographies even now include information about non-first impressions and anthology appearances shows how hard it has been to break away completely from the tradition of listing only what would interest collectors of firsts. Yet both non-firsts and anthology appearances may have textual significance, and both may be important in the history of a writer's reputation (anthologies sometimes carry more influence than any other form in which an author's work appears); surely they would have been more readily accepted into bibliographies if it had not been for the strength of collectors' preferences for firsts and the established practice of tailoring bibliographies to those preferences. If textual scholarship has been a principal force helping to move the descriptive bibliography of modern books beyond this limited concept, one should not therefore make the mistake of thinking that descriptive bibliography is essentially a tool for textual, or literary, work. Most advances made in descriptive bibliography have resulted in more details being put on record and thus move in the direction of bibliography as an end in itself—that is, as an historical study presenting facts of interest in their own right. What I suggested earlier about analytical bibliography can be said equally of descriptive bibliography: the more it is pursued as an independent activity, applicable to all kinds of books, whether literary or not, from all periods, the more it will establish a reliable historical context for the examination of any given book, or class of books.

III

These brief assessments of what has taken place in analytical and descriptive bibliography in this century can be no more than cursory surveys. But in isolating some of the main lines of development they can perhaps serve as background for considering what lies ahead. Analytical and descriptive bibliography are ultimately, of course, so interrelated that it seems artificial to treat them separately. They have to some extent had separate histories: published studies have tended to concentrate on either the analytical or the descriptive aspects of a bibliographical problem. Bowers's *Principles* limits itself to description but recognizes, and states explicitly, that analytical bibliography "must always precede description" (p. 364).

Clearly one cannot describe an edition, classifying its various issues, states, and impressions, without having employed all available analytical techniques, and applied them to as many copies as possible (copies which may appear to be "duplicate" but which cannot be finally considered duplicate until after such analysis has proved them to be). What has served over the years to demonstrate this relationship is textual study, for the most enlightened editors, from McKerrow onward, have recognized that a concern with an author's words cannot be divorced from a concern with the physical means of the transmission of those words. Although physical facts do not solve all textual cruxes, they set limits on what editors can speculate about. Critical editing—in which an editor makes emendations in a basic text—must always involve the editor's informed, but nevertheless subjective, judgment. But that judgment can only begin to operate after the demonstrable physical facts have been established.

The great outpouring of careful editions in the past quarter-century has followed in the wake of Greg's "The Rationale of Copy-Text," delivered at the English Institute in 1949.[30] But that influential statement, like Bowers's *Principles* at practically the same time, evolved from what had gone before—in this case, McKerrow's *Prolegomena for the Oxford Shakespeare* (1939) and Greg's own *The Editorial Problem in Shakespeare* (1942, 1951). The principal developments in editorial theory in this century have been made by persons who were also doing pioneer work in analytical and descriptive bibliography, first in connection with Shakespeare and his contemporaries and then with later literature. The large projects for editing American writers, begun in the 1960s under the CEAA, have provided the most dramatic recent demonstration of the interdependence of analytical and descriptive bibliography and editing.[31] Having behind them the precedent of six decades' work in Renaissance literature, they recognize the importance of bibliographical research in editing; but because very little of that bibliographical work had already been done for nineteenth-century American authors, it had to be undertaken by the editors of these volumes. The result shows the value and the naturalness of conducting all this research as related parts of a single program. Both the editions and the bibliographies (many of which are to be published in conjunction with the editions) are the better for this joint effort: textual decisions must rest on a knowledge of the publishing history of a work, as provided by the analysis and classification involved in description; and that process of description will itself be more thorough and accurate if it can draw on the results of the textual collations basic to editing. Indeed, it will be hard in the future to excuse descriptive bibliographers from engaging in collation of texts, for textual differences are physical differences and are logically a part of the evidence for description.

If there is one predominant point that twentieth-century physical bibliography has focused on and demonstrated, it is the interrelatedness between texts as intellectual constructions and the physical means by which they are transmitted. Determining just what words and punctuation a writer intended a text to consist of must begin with a knowledge of the physical history of the documents preserving that text, including any variations among copies of individual impressions. Anyone seriously interested in trying to understand what a text means, therefore, must start by questioning the reliability of the particular edition being used. Despite the efforts of the twentieth-century bibliographers, too many readers still do not understand that for any work of any period the conditions of its printing may affect the content of its text. The progress of twentieth-century bibliography has further shown that the analysis of the printing of any individual volume will benefit from the accumulation of details about contemporary printing practice derived from as wide an examination as possible of all kinds of books, whether literary or not. It is obvious, in turn, that all kinds of texts, whether literary or not, are affected by their physical transmission and are equally deserving of bibliographical investigation.

One can understand why literary works have provided the principal occasion for the development of physical bibliography. But it is time to recognize that all printed texts are subject to the vicissitudes of the printing process—and high time to dismiss the illogical notion that the nuances of "literary" works demand an attention to textual matters (both words and punctuation) not necessary for other kinds of works. Not only is it impossible to define exactly where "literature" leaves off and other writing begins; but readers of any piece of writing, if they are serious, will wish to have as much evidence as possible about what the author intended to say. One of the most encouraging signs of recent years is the editorial attention being devoted to so-called "nonliterary" writers like philosophers and scientists: volumes have already been published in comprehensive editions of Dewey, Locke, and William James, and editorial work is under way on Darwin and Einstein, among others. It has long been recognized that descriptive bibliography is important in helping to settle questions of priority in scientific nomenclature; but what must come to be more understood is that the very meaning of scientific texts is at stake. Inevitably the bibliographical and editorial scholarship directed toward belletristic texts will eventually be applied to all kinds of texts, and the sooner this expansion takes place the better for everyone concerned. Although Sir William Osler would probably not be drawn to some of the tasks now incumbent on bibliographers, he would unquestionably be in sympathy with the larger ends to be achieved by bibliographical cooperation among those working in different fields, and he would recognize that collecting and scholarship go hand in hand. There could be no better way to commemorate the first half century of his library than if the anniversay proceedings marked the beginning of a new era in the bibliographical and editorial treatment of scientific literature.

Notes

1. Francis, "The Bibliographical Society: A Sketch of the First Fifty Years," in *The Bibliographical Society 1892-1942: Studies in Retrospect* (London: Bibliographical Society, 1945), p. 16.

2. In the introduction to Osler's *Incunabula Medica*, published by the Bibliographical Society in 1923. A brief treatment of Osler as bibliographer also appears in John F. Fulton, *The Great Medical Bibliographers: A Study in Humanism* (Philadelphia: University of Pennsylvania Press, 1951), pp. 75-79.

3. This paper is quoted by Harvey Cushing in *The Life of Sir William Osler* (Oxford: Clarendon Press, 1926), II, 81-82.

4. "The Library School in the College," in *Report of the Directors and Inaugural Address, Summer School of Library Service, Aberystwyth* (Aberdeen: University Press, 1917), p. 35.

5. These ideas are also expressed in my essay on "The State of Bibliography Today," *Papers of the Bibliographical Society of America*, 73 (1979), 289-304.

6. On Bradshaw, see G. W. Prothero, *A Memoir of Henry Bradshaw* (London, Kegan Paul, Trench, 1888); on Proctor, see A. W. Pollard's memoir prefaced to Proctor's *Bibliographical Essays* (London: Chiswick Press, 1905). Also see Victor Scholderer, "Early Printed Books," in *The Bibliographical Society 1892-1942*, esp. pp. 32-36.

7. See Michael Sadleir, "The Development During the Last Fifty Years of Bibliographical Study of Books of the XIXth Century," in *The Bibliographical Society 1892-1942*, esp. pp. 146-53.

8. See Simon Nowell-Smith, "T. J. Wise as Bibliographer," *Library*, 5th ser., 24 (1969), 129-41.

9. The best discussion of the history of analytical bibliography is F. P. Wilson's "Shakespeare and the 'New Bibliography,'" in *The Bibliographical Society 1892-1942*, pp. 76-135—reprinted as a separate volume (Oxford: Clarendon Press, 1970), revised and edited by Helen Gardner. This period of bibliographical history has also been briefly treated by a distinguished medical librarian, F. N. L. Poynter, in *Bibliography: Some Achievements & Prospects* (Berkeley and Los Angeles: University of California School of Librarianship, 1961), esp. pp. 4-12.

10. "On Certain False Dates in Shakespearian Quartos," *Library*, 2nd ser., 9 (1908), 113-31, 381-409.

11. *Transactions of the Bibliographical Society*, 12 (1911-13), 213-318.

12. Some further discussion of McKerrow's book along these lines occurs in my review of Philip Gaskell's *A New Introduction to Bibliography* in *Costerus*, n.s. 1 (1974), 129-50.

13. "Elizabethan Spelling as a Literary and Bibliographical Clue," *Library*, 4th ser., 4 (1923-24), 1-8.

14. For something more on the Sadleir circle, see *Book Collecting: A Modern Guide*, ed. Jean Peters (New York: Bowker, 1977), pp. 212-14.

15. Bowers, "Notes on Running-Titles as Bibliographical Evidence," *Library*, 4th ser., 19 (1938-39), 315-38; Bowers, "The Headline in Early Books," *English Institute Annual 1941*, pp. 185-205; Hinman, "New Uses for Headlines as Bibliographical Evidence," *ibid.*, pp. 207-22; Bond, "Imposition by Half-Sheets," *Library*, 4th ser., 22 (1941-42), 163-67; Greg, *The Variants in the First Quarto of KING LEAR* (London: Bibliographical Society, 1940), pp. 40-57.

16. One useful example of the use of this kind of evidence is Robert K. Turner, Jr., "Reappearing Types as Bibliographical Evidence," *Studies in Bibliography*, 19 (1966), 198-209.

17. A brilliant instance of such analysis is Fredson Bowers, "An Examination of the Method of Proof-Correction in *Lear*," *Library*, 5th ser., 2 (1947-48), 20-44.

18. For example, "Observations on the Incidence and Interpretation of Press Figures," *Studies in Bibliography*, 3 (1950-51), 171-205; and "Bibliography and the Editorial Problem in the Eighteenth Century," 4 (1951-52), 41-55. Other important articles of Todd's appeared in other periodicals— such as "Press Figures and Book Reviews as Determinants of Priority," *Papers of the Bibliographical Society of America*, 45 (1951), 72-76, and "Concurrent Printing," 46 (1952), 45-57.

19. "Half-Sheet Imposition of Eight-Leaf Quires in Formes of Thirty-Two and Sixty-Four Pages," *Studies in Bibliography*, 15 (1962), 274-78; "A Note on Half-Sheet Imposition in Nineteenth and Twentieth Century Books," *Gutenberg Jahrbuch 1962*, pp. 545-47; "On the Imposition of the First

Edition of Hawthorne's *Scarlet Letter*," *Libarary*, 5th ser., 17 (1962), 250-55; "Evidence of Plate Damage as Applied to the First Impressions of Ellen Glasgow's *The Wheel of Life*," *Studies in Bibliography*, 16 (1963), 223-31.

20. The CEAA/CSE editions commented on briefly below, near the end of Part II and in Part III.

21. "Printers of the Mind: Some Notes on Bibliographical Theories and Printing-House Practices," *Studies in Bibliography*, 22 (1969), 1-75.

22. "New Uses of Watermarks as Bibliographical Evidence," *Studies in Bibliography*, 1 (1948-49), 151-82; "Watermarks Are Twins," 4 (1951-52), 57-91; "Chain-Indentations in Paper as Evidence," 6 (1954), 181-95. See also "Paper as Bibliographical Evidence," *Library*, 5th ser., 17 (1962), 197-212.

23. *Transactions of the Bibliographical Society*, 9 (1906-8), 31-52. This paper was followed (on pp. 53-65) by another influential discussion, Falconer Madan's "Degressive Bibliography."

24. *Library*, 2nd ser., 8 (1907), 193-217.

25. *Oxford Bibliographical Society Proceedings and Papers*, 1 (1922-26), 55-64.

26. "A Formulary of Collation," *Library*, 4th ser., 14 (1933-34), 365-82.

27. In the same year appeared *Standards of Bibliographical Description* (Philadelphia: University of Pennsylvania Press, 1949), a collection of three essays, by Curt F. Bühler, James G. McManaway, and Lawrence C. Wroth, each taking up a different class of material.

28. Most notably "Bibliography Revisited," *Library*, 5th ser., 24 (1969), 89-128.

29. I have surveyed in more detail two groups of bibliographies in "The Descriptive Bibliography of American Authors," *Studies in Bibliography*, 21 (1968), 1-24, and in "The Descriptive Bibliography of Eighteenth-Century Books," in *Eighteenth-Century English Books Considered by Librarians and Booksellers, Bibliographers and Collectors* (Chicago: Association of College and Research Libraries, 1976), pp. 22-33; I have also contributed a brief survey of bibliographies in general to *Book Collecting: A Modern Guide*, ed. Jean Peters (New York: Bowker, 1977), pp. 234-48.

30. *Studies in Bibliography*, 3 (1950-51), 19-36; reprinted in Greg's *Collected Papers*, ed. J. C. Maxwell (Oxford: Clarendon Press, 1966), pp. 374-91.

31. A listing of these editions, along with a survey of the literature on editing, can be found in the Modern Language Association of America's pamphlet *The Center for Scholarly Editions: An Introductory Statement* (New York: Modern Language Association of America, 1977), pp. 4-15 (printed also in *PMLA*, 92 [1977], 586-97).

Medical Historians,
Librarians and Bibliographers:
Will They Ever Meet?

Eric J. Freeman

Eric J. Freeman

It is widely believed (particularly by those who take no part in it) that scholarly study and research is an open, co-operative and cumulative process which adds inexorably to the total available sum of knowledge. The stock metaphor of "pushing back the frontiers of research" expresses precisely this popular view.

Reality is otherwise. In the sciences and the humanities probably just about as much knowledge is either forgotten or discarded as is newly won. What was knowledge in the past does not necessarily remain for ever accessible. It must often be won back hardly, or may even be lost for ever. Scholars are much like other men in allowing their small jealousies and personal shortcomings to delay or obscure truth. Their activities are often fragmented because of failures in communication, cultural myopia or linguistic isolation. Teaching and research in an institutional setting may be divided by disciplinary boundaries maintained sometimes from motives less than worthy.

The general truth of this somewhat gloomy view of scholarship may be exemplified, to an extent, from the particular instance of studies in the history of medicine. It will be the major theme of this essay that medical historians, librarians and bibliographers have so far shown little evidence of profiting from each other's skills and insights in a fruitful and sufficient manner. To demonstrate this sad state of affairs it is convenient to begin by looking at the place of the book in medicine and the consequent importance of bibliography in that context. An attempt will be made to outline a possible social history of the medical book and some consideration given to the role and responsibilities of the librarian in all these endeavours.

In the western world medicine has been an intensely bookish profession since at least the Middle Ages. Perhaps only among the lawyers has the book played such a central and controlling role in forming and preserving patterns of professional thought and education. The establishment of medicine as one of the higher faculties in the medieval universities led inevitably to the production of textbooks according to broad, general types. Hand in hand with the canon lawyers, the medieval doctors invented the textbook for students in essentially the form it still has today. An example is Guy de Chauliac's great book of surgery. Written in 1363, it was proliferated in more than thirty extant manuscripts, and thereafter printed in many editions, versions and translations. The book's traditional title describes it as an "Inventorium" or "Collectorium", terms which have aptly characterised textbooks of all ages. It begins with the author's justification for yet another textbook, continues with a not wholly accurate historical introduction, and then treats of the parts of the surgeon's craft in logical order adapted to facilitate learning. All of this is very familiar. The subject matter may be quaint to the modern mind but in shape and spirit is it so different (even down to the casual references) from almost any modern textbook of medicine or surgery? Predictably, it became out of date and no longer the last word in medical knowledge long before it ceased to be used; yet another recognisably modern mark of the textbook tribe. Even in size and weight Guy's book is comparable to a modern medical textbook.

More to the point than mere shape and internal arrangement, is the central role that the book has played and perhaps still plays in the transmission of medical authority and orthodoxy. Because of the awesome nature of his responsibilities in terms of human life and suffering the young doctor is rightly restricted within the boundaries defined by the authoritative statements of his trade for a much longer period than most professional journeymen. During his education, is any other kind of pupil than the medical student quite so liberally supplied with such a profusion of cribs, compendia, mnemonics, model answers, short-cut explanations of diagnoses and quick guides to treatment, all in book form? Again, perhaps only the lawyer. It is worth remembering that, in a period of contracting retail outlets, the medical profession is still able to support flourishing specialist bookshops.

In spite of computers and instrumental gadgetry, medicine is still a book dominated subject, producing and absorbing huge quantities of textbooks, specialist monographs and periodicals. For a long time the book has been a force powerfully shaping the traditional view of medicine as a learned profession and a potent symbol in the medical imagination which may not be ignored. In Osler's view, "the mind of medicine is illustrated in its literature, written and printed".[1]

This granted, one would expect a certain preoccupation with the medical book on the part of medicine's historians. Indeed, we may find medical historians paying close attention to the book; but as *raw material* rather than as *subject*. To a large extent, medical historians have looked upon manuscript and printed books primarily as information packages, rather than as objects which, singly and collectively, may be worthy of study in their own right.

This scholarly concentration on the book as *source*, rather than as *subject*, has had damaging effects on medical history as an academic discipline. Sound historical scholarship must proceed from a basis of solidly established sources of evidence. In preferring the glamour of interpretation *prior* to the establishment of textual foundations, historians of medicine have committed the classic error of putting the cart before the horse.

The bald assertion that the medical book has been neglected by historians is guaranteed to raise sceptical eyebrows in certain quarters. Medical historians will reply indignantly that there has been too much emphasis on bibliography, and in particular an obsession with the first editions of the great books of famous men, prized for their rarity and associations. The stern intellectual lineaments of medical thought and its all-important social context were neglected, they will tell you, in favour of the pernickety and expensive gossip of a book-collecting coterie. The names of William Osler and John Fulton may be uttered darkly as being among the more pernicious of this heretical sect. This view is exaggerated, uncharitable and unfair, but it contains an element of truth. Until the 1950s and 1960s there was indeed a predominant fashion in medical history for stories of great men and great books retailed in an anecdotal style little concerned with the broader perspectives of social history. This fashion is not to be laid solely at the door of the book collectors and amateur bibliographers, since it was a large element in the work of professional historians like Charles Singer and George Sarton.[2]

In advocating the study of the medical and scientific book it is convenient to consider two particular kinds of bibliographical investigation. The first is analytical bibliography, usually (but unfortunately not always) regarded as a necessary propaedeutic to textual study. Dr. Tanselle's lucid review if its long and honourable history of scholarly achievement renders unnecessary any further description or definition of analytical bibliography at this point.[3]

The other kind of bibliography has only recently begun to be attempted; the study of the book—its production, distribution and influence—as a social force. What one might refer to a little pompously as the "historical sociology of the book". Neither kind of bibliography—the book as a physical object nor the book as a social artifact—has thus far received much attention from historians of science and medicine, to the notable detriment of those subjects.

85

The sociology of the book is a late arrival on the bibliographical scene. There have been attempts to treat books and book production as factors in social structure and social change, or at least studies which tended towards that end. Straight histories of the book trade—of printing, publishing and bookselling—almost inevitably make some mention of the impact of the book upon society, or on the way some societies got the books they deserved.

The most general and influential study of books produced in the British Isles during the early centuries of printing is probably H.S. Bennett's three volumes on *English Books and Readers*, between 1475 and 1640.[4] Bennett's work was based on the *Short-Title Catalogue* by Pollard and Redgrave, the scope of which fixed his chronological limits. Bennett's sub-title ". . . a study in the history of the book trade from Caxton to . . . the reign of Charles I" promises far less than his final achievement. Each volume surveys the output of printers and publishers during a particular sub-division of his period, and includes some particularization of books in medicine and science. Bennett also looked at the general cultural background of book production, "the ways in which authors obtained a hearing, and the size and nature of the reading public". Deservedly popular and influential as they have been, Bennett's volumes remain essentially as he himself described them: ". . . my survey of the demand and supply in the book trade". Only occasionally (although frequently in a most stimulating manner) was he able to break out of the confines of internalist book trade history.

More sociological in both motivation and method than Bennett's work is Richard D. Altick's *The English Common Reader*, published in 1957.[5] Sub-titled "A social history of the mass reading public, 1800-1900", Altick's book has been popular, particularly in the English Literature departments of British and North American universities. In the growth of an industrial mass reading public Altick sees the formation of what seemed to him to be "a revolutionary social concept: that of democracy in print". The different emphasis of his book compared with Bennett's may be judged from the fact that only two of Altick's sixteen chapters deal directly with the book trade.

Religion, utilitarianism, education and literacy are some of the major social topics which Altick seeks to illuminate through a close study of what the ordinary man and woman read. That medicine and science figure hardly at all in this book is a measure both of its incompleteness and of its author's preoccupation with the growth of a new political force. Medical literature, popular or otherwise, rarely concerned itself with questions of democracy. As a pattern and exemplar *The English Common Reader* could prove fruitful to the attentive medical historian. He might care to reflect on the flourishing popular, not to say underground, medical literature which has been a feature of the western world since at least the seventeenth century. Popular herbals of the Culpeper kind, almanacks, books of household hints and recipes, chapbooks, laymen's guides to health and beauty would be his sources.[6] The literature of English "common medicine" is an extensive, largely unexplored, world of self-help and home therapy, employed by most of the people for most of the time, and far removed from the medicine of the textbooks and the Royal Colleges.

One other example of the social history of the book must suffice for present purposes. In 1958 some excitement was aroused by the publication in Paris of a book entitled *L'Apparition du livre*, initiated by one of France's foremost historians, Lucien Febvre and completed by his hardly less distinguished pupil Henri-Jean Martin.[7] The tradition of French historiography to which these two scholars belong is the intellectually fashionable "Annales" school which takes its name from the title of a prestigious journal, founded in 1929 by Marc Bloch and Febvre himself. Not surprisingly, the excitement transferred itself to the English-speaking world when the book was translated and published in 1976 as *The Coming of the Book: The Impact of Printing 1450-1800.*[8] Expectations were justifiably high. Here, at last, was the first full-scale social history of the book in the western world, informed and illuminated by all the special techniques of the "Annales" method; comparative history at its best, drawing data and wisdom from economics, sociology, anthropology, geography and so on.

In the event, *The Coming of the Book* proved a disappointing anticlimax. It is not a bad book in the sense of being inaccurate or misinformed or otherwise perverse. Much of it (in spite of the authors' and publisher's claims) is straight book-trade and printing history, chiefly valuable for reminding English-speaking students that France was so much more important in the book world, for so much longer, than Great Britain. (In fact it is neither comprehensive nor up to date as regards British affairs.) Only in the final chapter—"The book as a force for change"—does some originality of treatment reveal itself, yielding useful implications for anyone ambitious to explore the social history of the medical book in particular.[9]

What major themes may we anticipate in the so far unwritten social history of the medical and scientific book? We know very little about the ways in which medical knowledge was diffused in the centuries before our own. How, for example, did a seventeenth or eighteenth century country doctor, living in a provincial town, receive news of books lately published in the metropolis? What evidence is there that medical men in that isolated situation either required or sought such information? At least during the eighteenth century, there were elaborate business arrangements by which books published in London might be ordered by country dwellers through local booksellers, a function apparently taken over during the following century by wholesale booksellers located in the City. It is also clear that provincial bookseller/publishers were sometimes involved financially in the otherwise centralised publishing of the capital cities of London, Edinburgh and Dublin.[10] Febvre and Martin's observations on the spread of new commercial publishing and sales methods in the seventeenth and eighteenth centuries may be relevant here.[11] Quasi-national bibliographies began a sporadic existence in England in 1657, a little earlier in France. Their impact, if any, on the spread of medical knowledge needs investigation.

Until the nineteenth century Britain (with the partial exception of eighteenth century Scotland) was a medical backwater. The centres of concentration on the study of medicine and medical education were elsewhere on the continent of Europe. To keep up with the latest medical theories and events British doctors must have obtained and read continental books.

What is known of the international trade in medical and scientific books in the centuries between the fifteenth and the nineteenth? The so-called Latin trade in imported scholarly books has yet to be studied in much detail. Did the various post-Reformation attempts to limit or prevent the importation of foreign books affect medicine and science? If not, why? If they did, it would be good to know how, and to what extent, the restrictive legislation was circumvented.

Latin was the usual language of medicine until perhaps the seventeenth century, and in some places and for some purposes a great deal longer. Studies are needed of post-Renaissance medical and scientific Latin,

both to aid interpretation and to assist the translation of texts for the benefit of future generations of Latinless students. We also need to know why
and how the vernaculars intruded into the domain of Latin; some hard
socio-linguistic and educational facts to substitute for our current vague and
easy assumptions about the cultural consequences of European
nationalisms.

The relationships, business and otherwise, between medical authors
and their publishers have yet to be explored, although sources of information must surely exist. Literary studies provide some fine models; for example, of Michael Sadleir's work on Anthony Trollope and his publishers,[12] or
of John Butt and Kathleen Tillotson's study of *Dickens at Work*.[13]

It is received bibliographical wisdom that a major difference between
eighteenth and nineteenth century publishing was the predominance, in the
earlier century, of small, syndicated publisher/printer/booksellers, in contrast to the later rise of large, specialist publishers, some of whom concentrated on medicine.

The effects of this development on medical publishing, on the access
by doctors to their readers, professional and lay, together with the contrary
influence which the acceleration of medical research may have had on publishing patterns, are topics worthy of attention by historians. Related
research might profitably look at the origins and rise of the publisher's
reader, and of the referee system. The latter is now a standard feature of all
scholarly publishing, monograph or periodical. The system of submitting
manuscripts for a referee's opinion must have origins, and the suspicion is
that these may lie in medicine and science rather than in the humanities.

Such might be the staple of the social history of the medical book, if
only the historians would re-order some of their priorities. The dependence
of medicine and science upon the book *demands* investigation.

At this point an apparent paradox must be resolved. It has been ar-
gued that medical historians have neglected the social history of the medical
book. In apparent contradiction one may maintain that certain social
historical fashions current among medical historians have diverted attention from another, even more basic, kind of bibliography; analytical
bibliography as a tool for textual studies. In fact there is no logical conflict
between the two assertions. The social historical approach to medical history is not *necessarily* incompatible with bibliography and textual studies. It
is merely that too exclusive a preoccupation with social history *may* pro-

duce a scholarly tradition accidentally inimical to textual studies. This has surely happened at the present time.

Medical historians will admit, if pressed on the matter, that manuscripts, and printed books of the fifteenth, sixteenth and seventeenth centuries may present textual problems. This is understood to mean that they are likely to contain errors. It is commonly recognised, for example, that the pagination or foliation in early books is frequently, even usually, incorrect, while the more sophisticated understand that reference by signature is to be preferred for that reason. Very occasionally one meets an awareness that books of the hand-press period were sometimes corrected or otherwise altered during the printing process, and that consequently copies from the same edition will vary from each other.

Even such primitive bibliographical alarm bells become muffled and finally silenced when the medical historian reaches the late eighteenth, nineteenth and twentieth centuries. Perhaps they are deceived by the apparent modernity of books printed on wove paper with neo-classic typeface designs. The idea that twentieth century books in particular may offer textual problems (proofing errors apart) arouses alarm and despondency, even flat disbelief.

Certain bibliographical myths show a remarkable power of survival. Consider the following propositions, none of which would be difficult to exemplify from the medical historical writing of the past thirty years:-

1. The invention of printing *necessarily* introduced a new degree of accuracy and stability into learned communication.

2. The printed book enabled the same message to be duplicated *without important variation*.

3. The printed book was *always and necessarily* more accessible and cheaper than the manuscript codex.

4. Edition size and frequency of republication are *necessarily* an index of the public reception of a work.

5. The more recently a book has been printed the less likely it is to present substantial problems in the reconstruction of authorial intention.

6. An author's first printed editions necessarily and always have a canonical authority above any other source of his text—major revisions apart.

(This bibliographical half-truth is sometimes reinforced by the urge to seek out scientific priorities, origins and influences. In fact, priority of publication is rarely the most historically significant, or even the most interesting, feature of a new scientific or medical development.)

These common, and largely mistaken, assumptions are some of the more obvious examples of the conceptual traps into which the bibliographically unaware scholar can so easily fall.

Perhaps there is more at work here than merely a negative disregard of bibliographical techniques. Certain current historiographical fashions, heavily influenced by sociological and social history models, may have produced among medical historians a scholarly atmosphere unfriendly to bibliography. There may be some truth in the speculation that preoccupation with the social aspects of medicine in history has led to a devaluation of interest in the particular contributions of individual doctors and scientists. Medical historians are reluctant to encourage what they see as a sort of "cult of personality". Hence, emphases have changed radically from the study of, for example, William Harvey as an individual innovator making enduring contributions to "objective" science, to a preference for studies about Harvey as a seventeenth century general practitioner; Harvey as a Royalist, as an Aristotelean traditionalist, and so on.[14] A selection of recent titles from relevant journals will give something of the flavour of this now dominant historiographical emphasis: "Medicine, economy and science in 19th century America"; "Idealogy and medical abortion"; "Social and medical history: methodological problems in interdisciplinary quantitative research"; "Medical subculture in Victorian Lancashire"; "Child care, science and Imperialism: the contribution of social factors to the advance of medicalization in England". Powerful academic influences are encouraging young scholars to look beyond the individual for evidence of group activities and motives with which to characterise history in terms of structures, models, paradigms, oppositions and movements. Sometimes the historian's motives are explicitly ideological, producing explanations couched in terms of, say, economic determinism or the class struggle.

None of this is necessarily objectionable and implies no adverse reflection on the social history of medicine movement which has immeasurably improved the academic standards of the subject. But it is possible that, quite by accident, enthusiasm for social history has diverted attention from the importance of the text. Perhaps this is why, after so many years of dedicated effort from the thriving Harvey industry, there are as yet no satisfactory critical editions of his major printed works.

Compare the strikingly different situation in English literature studies. Literary historians and critics have found no difficulty in integrating social theories into their interpretation of literature and its history. At the same time the personality of the individual poet, novelist or dramatist has usually been acknowledged by a scholarly effort to produce definitive, critically edited, texts of their works. This has been the ideal, even if the achievement has fallen short. Analytical bibliography grew very largely out of literary studies. Bibliography's founding fathers—McKerrow, Greg, Bowers—as well as a host of other scarcely less bibliographically illustrious names, were either literary scholars or chose to work primarily on literary materials.

If it be important to use all the resources of analytical bibliography and textual criticism to reconstruct the authorial intentions of poets and novelists, surely it is no less an obligation to scholarship and high culture to do the same for the great works of science and medicine. But we look in vain for critically edited texts of most of the work of Vesalius, Paré, Harvey, Sydenham, Glisson, Boerhaave, Lind, Haller, Hunter, and a host of other lesser and greater names. What is particularly worrying is that one can detect little understanding that such a need exists.

Fredson Bowers, in a now famous short essay, had this to say about editions of nineteenth century American literature. His remarks are equally applicable to medical and scientific texts.

> The . . . problem is whether to edit the text critically or to content oneself with a reprint of some single document. Again, an argument cannot really exist in favor of a mere reprint, no matter how neatly such a procedure enables an editor to dodge his basic responsibility. It is probably safe to say that no nineteenth-century text of any length exists that is not in need of some correction, and possibly even of revisory emendation. Once an editor tinkers in any way with his original, he has entered upon the province of critical editing; and he had better go the whole way and be consistent than dip his big toe in the water and then draw back in alarm lest he suddenly find himself out of his depth.[15]

Medical historians have yet to show the slightest sign of getting their collective big toe wet in the waters of bibliography.

The feeble strengths and awful weaknesses in the present state of textual studies in science and medicine may be demonstrated from the history of one text of indisputable importance in the biological sciences—Charles Darwin's *On the Origin of Species by Natural Selection*. Students of Darwin begin with the advantage of possessing R.B. Freeman's splendid little book on the works of Charles Darwin, modestly but accurately sub-titled "An annotated bibliographical handlist".[16] Although not a full-scale analytical bibliography Freeman's book provides most of the essential information about editions and their relationships. Thus far Darwin has been well served.

At another level Darwin is also well, even superbly, served by Morse Peckham's variorum text of *On the Origin*.[17] In addition to printing all the variants, Peckham describes the process of composition, revision and publication, deals statistically with the variant readings, provides a very full descriptive bibliography, and even transcribes the publisher's records. A magnificent scholarly achievement—*but*, it is neither a critical edition of the *Origin* nor is it even an adequate substitute for such an edition. It remains essentially raw material for the editor's art.

In the first place Peckham's variorum text is unreadable. This is because it is a thesaurus of variants, not a continuous narrative. Second, and most fundamentally, it differs from a critical edition in that there is no exercise of the editor's critical judgement in the choice of readings. The reader is not provided with that clear perception of the author's original intentions, and revisions, which is the primary and distinguishing mark of the true critical edition. It is therefore no disparagement of Peckham's work to claim that it cannot take the place of the critical edition of the *Origin* that Darwin surely deserves.

Bibliographical innocence is fascinatingly demonstrated by one scholarly reaction to Morse Peckham's variorum text of the *Origin*. The reviewer in *Isis*, after pointing out that the book cannot be used for continuous reading, goes on to remark, with a deliciously unconscious irony—that "The ideal for such reading would be the reproduction of the six texts in six parallel columns, but this would be bulky and expensive."[18] It seems hardly necessary to comment on such a staggering unconcern for the fruits of three hundred years or more of textual and bibliographical scholarship.

Darwin's *On the Origin of Species* was chosen as a test case not only because of its undoubted importance, but also because it is a nineteenth century book. The weight of emphasis in historical medical research is already, and will be for the foreseeable future, firmly on the nineteenth and twentieth centuries. Out of any ten research students (supposing you can find so many in the history of medicine) seven of them will almost certainly be working on topics from this modern period. Yet it is precisely for these two centuries that bibliographical awareness among historians is at its lowest. It is not uncommon to find great skill and experience in archives and manuscript sources linked in the same researcher with a touching faith in the infallibility of the machine press.

Academic fashion may well be the most important factor discouraging scholars from editing medical and scientific texts, but there are undoubtedly other less intellectual reasons. Technical advances in reproduction processes and printing have created the current avalanche of reprints. In one form or another, and if expense is no object, it is now possible to get a copy of almost any book ever printed. Reprint publishing is very big business, absorbing the financial power and marketing skills of large, international companies.

Reprints have their obvious values and uses. Libraries (even well-heeled individuals) may make good gaps in their collections which would be impossible to fill from the regular antiquarian-book market. But in their present vulgar and undiscriminating profusion reprints may be an important factor inhibiting editorial ambitions. It is so easy to get photographic copies of all an author's editions, why bother with the editorial process?

There is, then, a gap between the bibliographers and the historians of medicine. The historians have failed to exploit either the wealth of information about the history of the book or the analytical techniques for the physical investigation of the book that several generations of bibliographers and textual critics have provided. The bibliographers (with some honourable exceptions) may be criticised in their turn for neglecting the medical and scientific book in favour of works of imaginative literature. (Incidentally, it is an odd tradition that excludes works of medicine and science from the realm of the imagination.)

What then of the librarians? What is their share of the blame for the present state of affairs.

Librarians, like farmers and publishers, will never admit that business is good. Everyone is chronically short of money and space. The rising prices of books and the falling values of currency have persuaded the profession to become account-watchers and budget-manipulators. Librarians can rarely be persuaded to count their blessings, even when these are considerable.

To all appearances libraries serving the history of medicine and science have made enormous progress in a remarkably short time. In Britain, Canada and the United States there are now collections in the history of medicine which either did not exist, or were undeveloped or inaccessible, only thirty or forty years ago. Catalogues, bibliographies and current awareness facilities exist today which were lacking as recently as the 1950s. There is no doubt that today's medical historians are vastly better off, at least so far as potential resources are concerned, than their fathers.

On the other hand, it is doubtful whether the growth of physical resources has been matched by an increase in the level of professional service and involvement. As librarians become more and more the (perhaps too willing?) victims of administrative growth and complexity, so have they tended to withdraw both from contact with library users and from personal involvement in scholarly subjects, such as medical history. Instead of living in symbiosis, librarians and scholars seem, too often, engaged in territorial competition, fighting each other for the possession of space, facilities and shrinking funds.

It is just those facilities that are meant as aids to the reader which most often deter him. Most scholars will admit to a hollow feeling of despair on encountering for the first time the catalogue hall of a strange library. The place bristles with monstrous card files, computer terminals, and enquiry desks whose staff seem to be perpetually at lunch. The hopeful reader is faced with a battery of so-called "aids" which effectively cut him off from the books he wishes to use.

Has librarianship become, to use Ivan Illich's devastating phrase, one of the "disabling professions"; whose principal aim is to convince the client that he is helpless without professional aid? A cautionary anecdote will illustrate the danger. At the end of this decade the British Library will be moved from its traditional home in Bloomsbury north to Somers Town. The preliminary announcement declared that the new building will have space for three and a half thousand readers and two and a half thousand staff![19]

Librarianship is not in essence a learned profession, despite the claims of the professional associations. It is primarily an administrative and clerical occupation whose individual practitioners may or may not be scholars. Librarians as such therefore have no special advantage within any scholarly field; except perhaps in that which deals with the history and physical construction of books. Here, if anywhere, the librarian ought to be able to take a lead and set examples because of the special nature of his professional training, situation and opportunities. Furthermore, librarians as bookmen, as well as (inevitably) administrators, ought to be able to provide that essential link between bibliography and the history of medicine and science.

Those librarians who by inclination and training favour the early period of printed books and who perhaps feel that anything written after 1700 barely qualifies as history, will have to readjust to a radically new set of values and priorities. It is matter for reflection that, for example, the library of the Wellcome Institute is making great efforts to complete its published series of catalogues of books printed up to 1850 at a time when (as mentioned above) the weight of emphasis in medical historical research is shifting from earlier periods onto the nineteenth and twentieth centuries. This represents a considerable investment of professional time, skills and, of course, money and is almost certainly being matched or surpassed at the National Library of Medicine and at other American and Canadian institutions. Even as librarians strive to bring the riches of the seventeenth and eighteenth centuries to the notice of scholars, the scholars themselves are turning more and more to modern periods. There is an irony here, the logical consequences of which we have yet squarely to face.

The early books cannot, of course, be abandoned. But it is time to think seriously about the collection and conservation of books and journals from the late nineteenth and the twentieth centuries, and it must be done quickly in spite of the squeaks and protests of accountants and administrators anxious about extra space and staff levels. The signs are clear for all to read. Sotheby's the London auctioneers have, perhaps for the first time ever, offered at auction considerable numbers of twentieth century medical books. Every shelf-discard from the medical libraries needs to be carefully checked without overmuch concern for the risks of acquiring ephemeral trash.

Thomas Bodley's librarian (so the story goes) threw out certain rather scruffy sixteenth and early seventeenth century pamphlets on the grounds that they were unworthy of a great academic library. His unregarded trifles were Shakespeare play quartos.

Will the historians, librarians and bibliographers ever meet? In other words, shall we see the special skills and insights of each group, combined in the service of the history of science and medicine? The omens are not good. Relatively few people are involved in these subjects, whether as historians, bibliographers or librarians, so that discussion tends to be narcissistic. Changes in general and professional education threaten to drive specialists apart rather than unite them. It is uncertain, for example, how much longer librarians educated in Great Britain will be taught anything at all about historical bibliography. A crippling loss affecting all three professions is the accelerating retreat of the classical languages from everyone's educational systems.

One thing is certain. If it be granted that the primary evidence for the history of medicine, as for all the other special histories, is contained for the most part in books, manuscript and printed, then it follows that a profound knowledge *of*, a sceptical respect *for*, and a scholarly obsession *with* the book, both as a physical object and as social phenomenon, must be the necessary prerequisites for a healthy, vigorous and solidly-based academic discipline.

Notes

1. *Incunabula Medica: A Study of the Earliest Printed Medical Books, 1467-1480* (London: The Bibliographical Society, 1923), p. 2.
2. For example, Sarton's *Six Wings: Men of Science in the Renaissance* (Bloomington, Ind.: Indiana University Press, 1957) and Singer's *Short History of Medicine Introducing Medical Principles to Students and Non-medical Readers* (Oxford: Clarendon Press, 1928), *A Short History of Biology: A General Introduction to the Study of Living Things* (Oxford: Clarendon Press, 1931), and *A Short History of Science to the Nineteenth Century* (Oxford: Clarendon Press, 1941).
3. See above pp. 56 to 79.
4. 3 vols. (Cambridge: University Press, 1952-1970). A second edition of volume 1 appeared in 1969.
5. (Chicago: University of Chicago Press, 1957) reprinted 1963.
6. For an excellent example of what might be achieved, although on a wider scale of reference than the purely medical, see Bernard S. Capp, *Astrology and the Popular Press. English Almanacs 1500-1800* (London: Faber, 1979).
7. (Paris: Albin Michel, 1958).
8. Translated by David Gerard, edited by Geoffrey Nowell-Smith and David Wootton (London: NLB, 1976).
9. Elizabeth Eisenstein's massive two-volume work, *The Printing Press as an*

Agent of Change: Communications and Cultural Transformations in Early-Modern Europe, 2 vols. (Cambridge: Cambridge University Press, 1978) arrived on the scene too late for consideration here. A rapid preliminary scan suggests that it may be an important general guide for the kind of particular studies outlined in this article.

10. On these matters see the standard account in Marjorie Plant, *The English Book Trade: An Economic History of the Making of Books*, 3rd ed. (London: Allen & Unwin, 1974) supplemented and modified by the relevant sections of Philip Gaskell, *A New Introduction to Bibliography* (Oxford: Clarendon Press, 1972).

11. Febvre and Martin, *The Coming of the Book*, p. 234 ff.

12. *Library*, 4th ser., 5 (1924-25), 215-242.

13. (London: Methuen, 1957).

14. A recent example is Jerome F. Bylebyl (ed.) *William Harvey and his Age. The Professional and Social Context of the Discovery of Circulation* (Baltimore and London: Johns Hopkins Press, 1979). Two of the contributions included, by Charles Webster and R.G. French respectively, are entitled, "William Harvey and the crisis of medicine in Jacobean England" and "The image of Harvey in Commonwealth and Restoration England".

15. "Some Principles for Scholarly Editions of American Authors", *Studies in Bibliography*, 17 (1964), 223-228.

16. 2nd ed. (London: Dawson, 1977).

17. (Philadelphia: University of Pennsylvania Press, 1959).

18. 51 (1960), 211.

19. *Library Association Record*, 80 (1978), 182.

The Contributors

Lloyd G. Stevenson is Director of the Institute of the History of Medicine at Johns Hopkins University, Baltimore.

Charles G. Roland is Jason A. Hannah Professor of the History of Medicine at McMaster University, Hamilton.

Richard J. Durling is a member of the Institut fur Geschichte der Medizin und Pharmazie der Christian-Albrechts-Universitat, Kiel.

Estelle Brodman was, until recently, Librarian and Professor of Medical History in the School of Medicine of Washington University, St. Louis.

G. Thomas Tanselle is Vice-President of the John Simon Guggenheim Memorial Foundation, New York.

Eric J. Freeman is Librarian of the Wellcome Institute for the History of Medicine, London.

Index

compiled by Peter Greig

(The letter "n" refers to the notes following each paper; for example, the reference "41n23" will be found on page 41, note 23)

manuscripts 32, 33, sociology of the
book 87-88
Francis, F.C.
on Osler and the Bibliographical
Society 57
Francis, William Willoughby 3,
Bibliotheca Osleriana editor 22
Freeman, Eric 4, 7
Freeman, R.B.
Darwin bibliography 93
Fulton, John F. 3, 4, 49, on
bibliography 7, Boyle bibliography
7, *The Great Medical Bibliog-
raphers* 3, on Keynes' biblio-
graphical form 19, and Osler 48,
85

GALEN: *De Inaequali Intemperie* 33,
De Rigore (*De Malitia Com-
plexionis*) 33, *Methodus Medendi*
(*De Ingenio Sanitatis*) 33
Gallup. Donald
T.S. Eliot bibliography 71-72
Garrison, Fielding
on Sudhoff 37
Gaskell, Elizabeth
Wives and Daughters 23
Gaskell, Philip
Baskerville bibliography 71, Foulis
Press bibliography 71
Gasquet, F.A. 15, 17
General Electric 51
George Dock Lecture on the History
of Medicine (1966) 21
Germany: manuscripts 32, 35
Gesamtkatalog der Wiegendrucke 52
Gesner, Conrad 3, 6
Gibson, Strickland
"Standard Descriptions of Printed
Books" 69
Great Britain 17, 23, 88,
manuscripts 31, 32, 35
sociology of the book 86-88
Greg, Walter W. 6, 17, 61, on
bibliography 11, *A Bibliography of
the English Printed Drama to the
Restoration* 69, on collation
formulas 69, *The Editorial Problem
in Shakespeare* 75, on the Pavier

quartos 62, 67, on proofreading 64,
"The Rationale of Copy-Text" 75,
"Some Points in Bibliographical
Descriptions" 68-69
Guy de Chauliac 83-84

HALLER, Albrecht von 3
Harvey, William
De Generatione 12, *De Motu
Cordis* 12, studies on 91, 92, 98n14
Hazen, Allen T.
Strawberry Hill Press bibliography
71, Walpole bibliography 71
Herbert, William 59
Hill, R.H.
Bibliotheca Osleriana editor 22
Hinman, Charlton J.K.
Hinman collator 72, *The Printing
and Proof-Reading of the First
Folio of Shakespeare* 11, 65, on
running-titles 64
Hippocrates
Aphorisms 33, *Prognostics* 33
HISTLINE 6-7, 52
history: and bibliography 3, 4, 5, 20-
21, 57, 73-74, author bibliography
7, 19-20, 60, 68, 70-73; and books
20, 57, 85-88; and medicine 4, 7,
31, 83, 93-94, 96-97; and Osler
12, 14; and publishing 4-6, 20, 57-
58, 62-77 passim, 85-90, medical
publishing 86-90 passim; and
Sadleir 70-71, 73
Holland, *see* Netherlands
Holland, Henry 23
Holland, Peter 23
Holmes, Oliver Wendell 14, *The
Guardian Angel* 22-23

IBERIA
manuscripts 35, *see also* Spain
incipits 34
incunabula 58-59, 66, 67
Index-Catalogue 6, 48, factory system
used 51, and Osler 12, 13
Index Medicus 3, 6, 51
Indiana Historical Society series 71
Institute for the History of Medicine,
Kiel 34